the eczema detox

About the author

Respected Australian nutritionist Karen Fischer is the author of five books including the award-winning The Healthy Skin Diet *and* The Eczema Diet, *which featured on prime time news as a 'breakthrough diet for eczema'. In private practice, Karen runs the Eczema Life Clinic in Sydney. Karen has two children, including her daughter who previously suffered from eczema.*

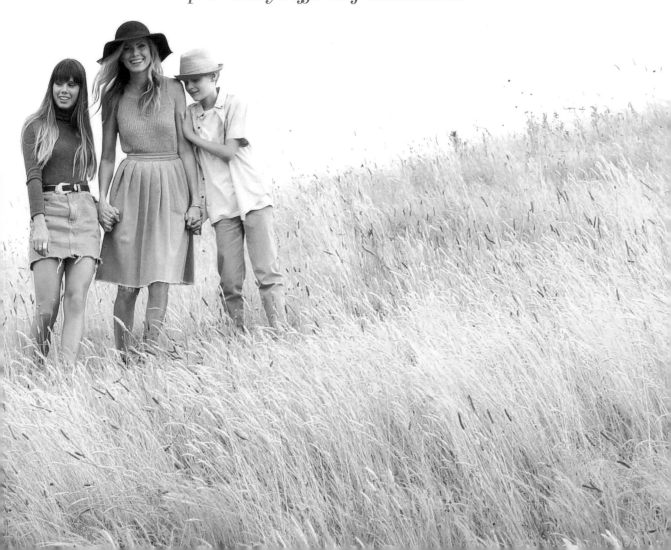

the eczema detox

the low-chemical diet for eliminating skin inflammation

KAREN FISCHER BHSc, Dip. Nut.

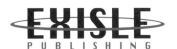

'This diet and the supplements are healing my eczema and changing my life. I feel pain- and itch-free for the first time in my life.'

RHIA, UNITED STATES

'Our daughter Georgie suffered from eczema and all she wanted was for the pain to go away. Doctors could not help her other than to say come back when you turn fifteen, you will grow out of it. For Georgie this was not an option. The eczema would start to bleed and she couldn't stand the pain and all she wanted to do was hide or die. So we made an appointment to see Karen. She placed Georgie on the eczema diet which also contained the Skin Friend product. After a few weeks we started to see an improvement in Georgie. It has now been eight months since Georgie started using the program and she is now leading a normal life and you wouldn't even know that she had suffered from eczema.'

KEITH, AUSTRALIA

'Being 57 years old and struggling with debilitating eczema on my hands for the first time in my life has been a source of deep discouragement. The past year has been spent in anguish and humiliation and franticly searching for relief. Allergist testing revealed nothing helpful. Countless creams and ointments and oils were expensive experiments and seemed futile. One day I ran across an article about *The Eczema Diet* and ordered the book that very hour ... I read about the Skin Friend supplements and ordered them as fast as I could get them! Following the diet and supplementations as carefully as I could, I actually started seeing some relief within a week. It's now several months later ... my hands are virtually free from their painful bondage and I can function and feel like a normal person again!'

GINGER, UNITED STATES

'Hello Karen, after seven long years suffering dermatitis herpertiformis and many visits to dermatologists and doctors with no improvement, I was happy to try your diet. For the first time in years I am nearly DH free and the hideous scars are healing!'

LORRAINE

'Please pass along a great big THANK YOU to Karen Fischer and all the Eczema Life team! I am finally seeing good healing after six months of struggling with intense eczema over all of my arms, chest and thighs. I have never had eczema like this in my entire life — I'm 62 — so this caught me by surprise.

Little by little I have improved. Now, at six months into the diet, I am adding even more foods and wearing short sleeves again! Your philosophy that it all begins in the liver was so accurate for me — and I'm sure others. Thank you so much for your work. I am thrilled to have my health back!'

QUIN, AUSTRALIA

'My breastfed baby started to get eczema at three months old (she's now six months). The doctors told me it was probably from soap or detergent and gave me a cream. After two weeks on the creams it looked just as bad as before. I became so frustrated and started to look into the fact that maybe what I was eating was to blame. This book was a lifesaver. It can be so overwhelming to try and start from scratch to figure out what's triggering your baby's eczema. Karen Fischer had all the research done for me, told me where to start and what foods to avoid. Within two weeks of following the book, my daughter's skin was so clear it was amazing!'

KRISTEN, UNITED STATES

'I am a 50-year-old female who has always remained fit and healthy but unfortunately have suffered from eczema and allergies my whole life. I must say I was very skeptical as I had tried *everything!* Well let's say it has changed my life; I'm not a religious person but it has become a Bible. By three weeks my skin was showing huge improvement and by six weeks my eczema had completely cleared up. Nothing short of a miracle! Now at five months I continue the diet, although not as strictly, and still take Skin Friend every day. I cannot thank you enough that I am eczema free!'

PAULA, AUSTRALIA

First published 2018

Exisle Publishing Pty Ltd
PO Box 864, Chatswood, NSW 2057, Australia
226 High Street, Dunedin, 9016, New Zealand
www.exislepublishing.com

Copyright © 2018 in text: Karen Fischer

Karen Fischer asserts the moral right to be identified as the
author of this work.

All rights reserved. Except for short extracts for the purpose
of review, no part of this book may be reproduced, stored in a
retrieval system or transmitted in any form or by any means,
whether electronic, mechanical, photocopying, recording or
otherwise, without prior written permission from the publisher.

A CiP record for this book is available from the National Library
of Australia.

ISBN 978-1-925335-53-8

Designed by Tracey Gibbs
Typeset in Abril and Miller Text
Printed in China

This book uses paper sourced under ISO 14001 guidelines from
well-managed forests and other controlled sources.

10 9 8 7 6 5 4 3 2 1

Disclaimer
This book is a general guide only and should never be a substitute
for the skill, knowledge and experience of a qualified medical
professional dealing with the facts, circumstances and symptoms
of a particular case. The nutritional, medical and health
information presented in this book is based on the research,
training and professional experience of the author, and is true
and complete to the best of their knowledge. However, this book
is intended only as an informative guide; it is not intended to
replace or countermand the advice given by the reader's personal
physician. Because each person and situation is unique, the
author and the publisher urge the reader to check with a qualified
healthcare professional before using any procedure where there
is a question as to its appropriateness. The author, publisher and
their distributors are not responsible for any adverse effects or
consequences resulting from the use of the information in this
book. It is the responsibility of the reader to consult a physician
or other qualified healthcare professional regarding their
personal care. This book contains references to products that
may not be available everywhere. The intent of the information
provided is to be helpful; however, there is no guarantee of
results associated with the information provided.

Photo credits
Copyright © in photographs Karen Fischer; except pp. ii, viii, ix, 103,
121, 179, 180, 222 copyright © in photographs Lyn McCreanor.
Cover image: Spelt Pancakes with Banana Nice Cream and Papaya
Nice Cream; ceramic plate and jug by Made of Australia.

Contents

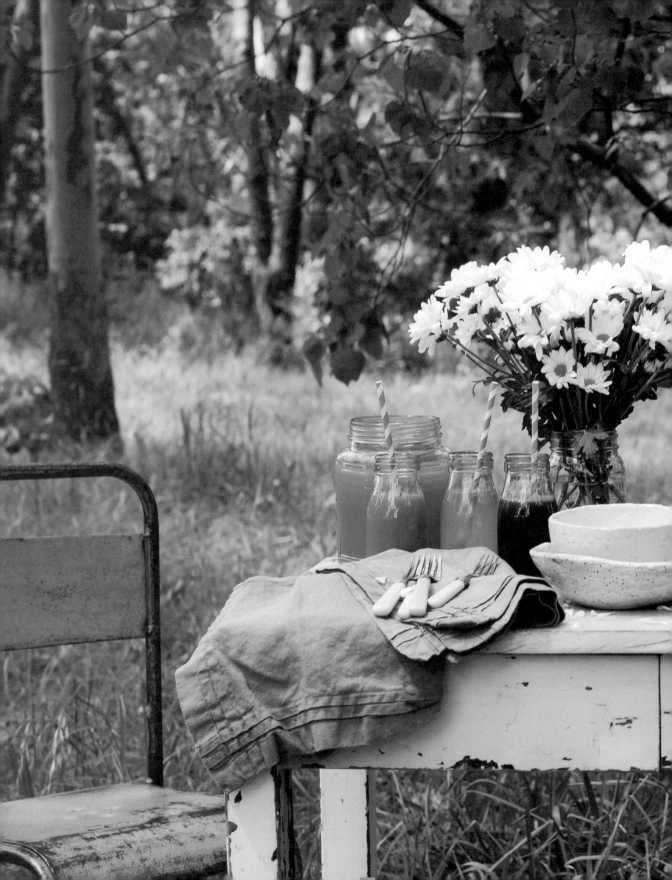

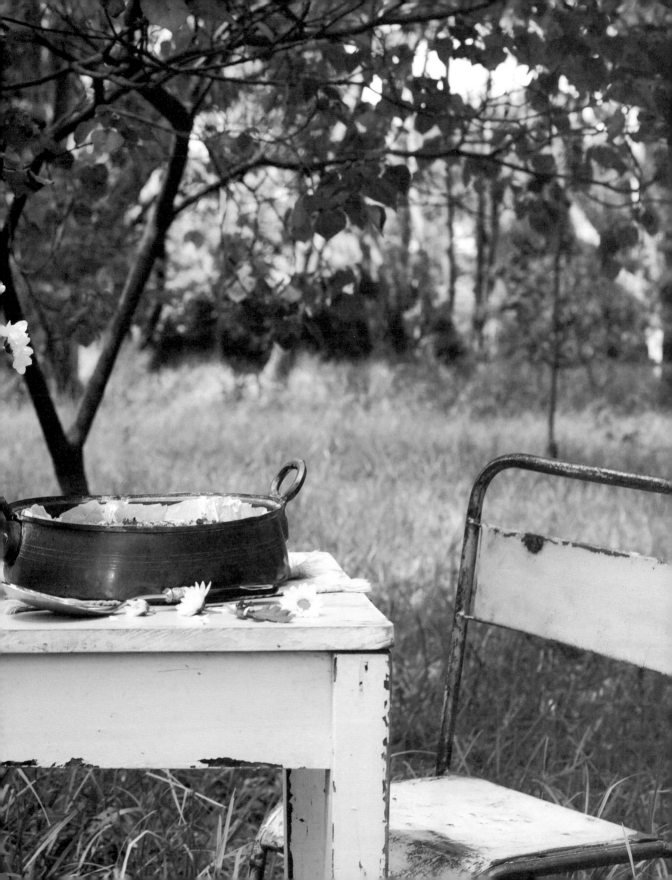

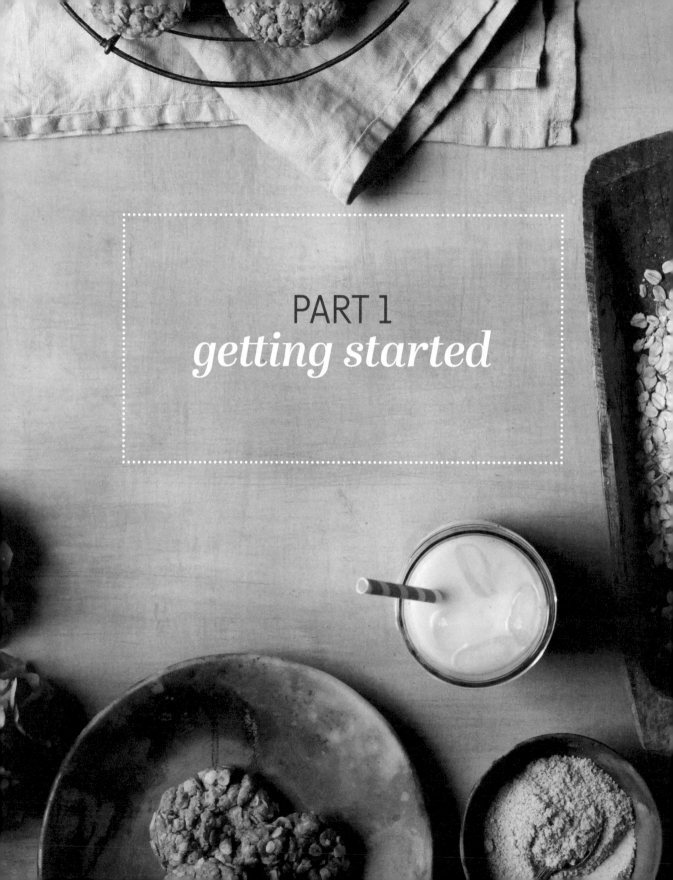

PART 1
getting started

Introduction

In my household we have one vegan, one pescatarian and one meat-eater who is sensitive to salicylates, dairy and soy. So I am right here with you. I know it can be difficult when a family member is first diagnosed with eczema and food sensitivities. I know what it's like to give up some of the foods you love because they are hurting you. Cooking is more of a chore than normal ... until you get the hang of it. However, as a result of making dietary changes, my family and I no longer suffer from skin disorders and my children are calmer and happier.

My own teenage years were a series of stressful and embarrassing events thanks to having a range of skin problems, including severe hand dermatitis. I was tired and irritable most of the time. However, unknown to me, the foods I was eating were to blame. I thought being healthy meant drinking close to a litre of milk daily plus eating bowls of flavoured yoghurt. I was a fussy child and I lived mostly on milkshakes, toast, and meat and three veg or spaghetti bolognese. I topped it off with ice-cream for dessert each night. Tea and chocolate (caffeine) gave me body aches. I was dairy intolerant and deficient in a range of nutrients, but I had no idea.

In my late twenties, a chemical exposure when I flea-bombed the house triggered psoriasis which spread to over half of my body. I was sensitive to chemicals. I later found out, after gargling aspirin and being rushed to hospital with a swollen throat, I was also sensitive to a chemical called salicylates. After many tests, my doctor suggested (several times) that I should eat healthier and exercise. I was sceptical at first. I need scientific proof, and lots of it, before I will go along with any health movement. So I studied to become a qualified nutritionist, then I completed a Health Science Degree, and read every diet and natural therapy book I could find, and I finally changed my diet. It was hard at first — I had never eaten salad before. However, my new-found energy was amazing and I had glowing, clear skin for the first time in my life.

During my studies I had a light bulb moment I'll never forget. While I was in nutritional biochemistry class I found a solution to my salicylate sensitivity. It not only fixed my sensitivity, it would eventually help my unborn child's eczema.

My daughter Ayva developed eczema when she was two weeks old. When she was ten months old, a nurse from the local early childhood centre who had seen her a few months earlier exclaimed, 'Has your child *still* got eczema?' I thought: what a rude comment, eczema is a genetic condition and *what could I do about it*? I was a nutritionist and I had not considered looking at treatment options for my baby beyond cortisone cream and thick ointments. As soon as the nurse mentioned Ayva might have 'salicylate sensitivity' a light bulb moment happened again. I thought: *I know how to fix that.*

As Ayva was under age one I did not begin with a supplement regime to reverse salicylate sensitivity. Instead, we followed a standard low-salicylate diet. Then one day Ayva, who was growing resentful about being different from her friends, ate some food at a friend's birthday party and her eczema returned on her arms, legs and face. Now her eczema would not budge. She was two years old and I thought it was time to design a diet routine for her that was both low in salicylates and healthy. The aim: make her body stronger and *less* sensitive to foods so she could eventually eat a wider variety of foods. To my surprise and excitement, two months later Ayva's skin looked beautiful and she no longer needed topical steroid creams.

Friends and family said Ayva had simply grown out of her eczema. I thought they might be right so I stopped the regime and Ayva's eczema returned. So I put her back on the program and once again her eczema cleared up. While it took time and patience, we eventually expanded Ayva's diet so she could eat a wide range of foods without her eczema returning. Best of all she was no longer sensitive to dust mites or walnuts, and she could pat our family cat and swim in chlorinated pools without her skin flaring up.

The Eczema Detox

What I am about to tell you in this book is probably vastly different to the advice you have read on the internet. In fact, some of my advice will be in direct conflict with what you believe is good for your skin. What you will find, however, is that this program is tailored to you and my advice is scientifically referenced so you can check the validity of the sources.

So if you have tried a range of healthy eating programs and you still have eczema, all I ask is *be open to trying something different*. I also suggest that you do not combine your current eczema program or nutritional supplement regime with this one as this could affect your results. If you need to complete your current health program before beginning this one, do so. See how it goes and then if you still have eczema, stop that regime and begin one of the programs in this book.

I want to make it clear that the programs in this book are not designed to temporarily suppress the symptoms, like an antihistamine drug. *Because when you suppress the body's cries for help (with drugs and natural potions), the symptoms will surface again and again, often in another form such as asthma or hay fever.* This switching of symptoms is called the 'atopic march'. So instead of relying on suppressants, use this book and do the detective work needed to find out what is irritating your skin. Then allow time for your body to heal from the inside out. If, at the end of the program, you still have some skin problems, refer to Chapter 12, 'FAQs and problem solving' (p. 112). It is sometimes necessary to do a little more detective work to see what foods might be continuing to cause issues.

I know you might be desperate to end the embarrassment and the frustration of skin irritations as quickly as possible, but be patient. Try the programs in this book for at least three months for best results.

Itchy kids can be fussy kids

If you have a child with eczema, encourage them to become a 'food detective' and document their 'itchy foods' and their 'happy foods' (ones that don't make them itchy). Make it a game. Encourage them to keep a Food Detective Diary so they are engaged in their own healing.

I know it can be hard to change a child's diet. My son is nine and strong willed. In fact, I had two of the world's fussiest eaters and if I can change their eating habits anyone can do it. If you are having trouble convincing a fussy eater to follow the program, I suggest reading *Healthy Family, Happy Family* (Exisle Publishing) as soon as you can, because it will bring the joy back into your meal times.

What about allergy testing?

If you have done food allergy testing that is great. It is a good start, but allergy testing is often incomplete and it cannot screen for chemical intolerances. Allergy tests can also be inaccurate as they often show the foods you eat the most, not the ones you are intolerant to. This book will show you how to get an accurate diagnosis of the foods you react to, so you'll know what to eat and what to avoid to become eczema-free.

Other skin inflammatory disorders

As this book can help other types of skin inflammation, including psoriasis, rosacea and topical steroid withdrawal, I will often refer to 'skin inflammation' or 'skin inflammatory disorder/s' instead of eczema. When I refer to 'eczema' it is usually because the scientific research was conducted on eczema patients. However, if you have another skin disorder the information is still relevant to you.

As everyone is different, there are three eczema programs to choose from: the Eczema Detox Program, the Food Intolerance Diagnosis (FID) Program and the Skin Supplement Program. Refer to Chapter 1 for more details.

Supplements

I truly believe people with stubborn skin disorders need extra help to boost their nutrient intakes. The reason they have eczema and other skin rashes in the first place is often triggered by undiagnosed nutritional deficiencies. These deficiencies are then masked with drugs, antihistamines and other suppressants. Skin inflammation and stress also deplete nutrients in your body and a regular healthy diet is often not enough to keep the skin clear. This may be due to poor digestion, genetics, fatty liver and other internal health issues. However, whatever the case, supplements can speed up the road to recovery.

In the past, my readers have said it was very difficult to find the right supplements. So they often bought the wrong products and had to buy many bottles at great expense. At the insistence of some of my patients who said, 'Make me the supplement that cleared up your daughter's skin', I began prescribing Skin Friend. And nearly a decade later, after years of testing the products, I have finally launched my own range of skin supplements to accompany my health programs. So please note that I recommend these supplements within this book, along with supplements that are not my own brand. I hope this makes following your chosen program from this book easier for you.

Note: if you are ill and/or taking prescribed medications, please check with your doctor before changing your diet or taking supplements.

Record your progress

Once your skin rash improves, it can be easy to forget how bad your skin inflammation was before. I had one lady call me after a month to complain that her child's skin had not improved. I checked his 'before' photo, which showed his back was practically covered in about thirty large red welts. His latest photos showed he had about twenty tiny red dots on his back. They were still itchy but their size and number had reduced remarkably. I advised his mother *it can take longer than a month to be eczema-free and to keep going as he was making fantastic progress.* I have included a 'before' and 'after' photo for you to see the progress that can be made — see p. 9.

It is useful to document your journey to clear skin. I recommend taking photos of your skin (or your child's skin) before you begin the program so you can keep track of your progress. Then take new photos each month for comparison.

Note: in order to keep this book short and to the point (so you can get started straight away) I have omitted information that I felt was more suitable for blog posts. So you'll see some places throughout the book where I suggest you visit my websites to access more information about a particular subject.

I wish you all the best and if you need extra information visit www.eczemalife.com and www.skinfriend.com. I also invite you to sign up to my newsletter and join our caring online community for extra support along your journey to clear skin. See 'Useful resources' on p. 220 for more information.

Thank you for putting your trust in me.
With love,
Karen Fischer

FAQs

'If I follow one of the programs in this book, how long will it take before my skin gets better?'

It might be only a matter of weeks if you have a new case of eczema, or many months, especially if you have suffered for decades with your skin problem. People who can commit fully to the program often find it works for them within eight to twelve weeks. The only way to know for sure is to begin and see for yourself.

A good rule to use when determining how long it might take you to clear up your skin disorder is this: for every year of illness it might take a month to heal. For example, if you have had eczema for the past ten years it may take up to ten months to be eczema-free; if you have had psoriasis for less than a year, you could be clear-skinned after a month. A one-year-old infant who recently developed eczema might look great in a week or two ... It also depends on your level of commitment to be a part of your own healing and follow the advice in this book.

I have seen people with severe life-long eczema who take several return consults and a year to completely heal their eczema, but the point is they *did* get better and they were absolutely thrilled with their new soft skin. You can do it too – it's a matter of identifying which foods and chemicals are *your* triggers, nourishing your body with nutrients and restoring optimal liver function. Some people work out their trigger foods with ease, while others need to switch programs and investigate further, but the point is to keep going until you get the relief you desire.

'What does it mean to "detox"?'

A regular 'detox' is a cleansing process where you abstain from a variety of unhealthy foods and drinks for a period of time in order to reduce the amount of toxins, saturated fats and dairy you consume. It usually involves consuming healthy detoxifying vegetable juices and alkalizing foods to improve the acid–alkaline balance in the body. While the Eczema Detox does this, it goes a step further in order to target skin inflammation.

The Eczema Detox reduces your intake of *natural* chemicals, including salicylates and amines, in order to give your liver a break from chemical overload. Chemical overload occurs when the amount of chemicals you consume exceeds the rate at which your liver is capable of detoxifying them. For example, the more chemicals you are exposed to (via skin care, cleaning products and your diet) the more vitamins and minerals you need to consume to help your liver detoxify these chemicals. The Eczema Detox is designed to correct these imbalances.

Chapter 1
Foods that bite: what is chemical intolerance?

'When in doubt, eat fruits and veggies.' Might seem like good advice except for the fact that fruits and vegetables contain all-natural phytochemicals known as salicylates. As with other plant foods that bite back, salicylates evolved to fight predators. Many people today are so salicylate intolerant that they experience adverse reactions not only to drugs but also to salicylate-rich foods like fruits and vegetables.[1]

DR WESTON A. PRICE

You may have heard of 'chemical sensitivity' or 'chemical intolerance'. If you are sensitive to chemicals you might adversely react to perfumes, household cleaning products and the chlorine in your pool. You are likely to be sensitive to food colourings, artificial flavourings and preservatives. Many health-conscious eczema sufferers avoid artificial additives and chemical cleaning products and believe they are living a low-chemical lifestyle. They might also avoid lactose from dairy — but they still have eczema. The reason the eczema persists can often be attributed to the *natural* chemicals in a person's diet. According to research conducted at the Royal Prince Alfred Hospital Allergy Unit in Sydney, people with eczema are most likely to react to a natural chemical called salicylates and, to lesser degrees, preservatives, food colourings, amines, nitrates, MSG and other glutamates.[2]

Salicylate intolerance (salicylate sensitivity)

Salicylates (pronounced suh-lis-a-lates) are natural pesticide chemicals produced by plants for self-protection. Organic fruits and vegetables, when attacked by pests, produce more salicylates as a deterrent. Salicylates also work as a natural preservative — so it's no wonder people adversely react to them! A normal healthy diet can contain up to 200 mg of salicylates, from foods such as tomato, avocado, citrus fruits, teas and nuts.[3] People with eczema and other skin inflammatory disorders often don't realize they are sensitive to salicylates and they can suffer for years as a result.

Salicylate sensitivity was first reported in 1902, when a patient ingested a new drug called aspirin (a salicylate medication) and experienced a life-threatening anaphylactic reaction and hives.[4] Asthma attacks triggered by salicylate ingestion were first reported in 1919, and several asthmatics died after ingesting aspirin in the 1920s (the lifesaving EpiPen had not yet been invented).[5] Then in the 1970s, Dr Ben Feingold discovered that salicylates in *foods* could make children hyperactive and his research confirmed that some children performed poorly at school as a result.[6] It wasn't until the 1980s that the link between salicylate sensitivity and eczema was confirmed by Australian researchers Loblay and Swain from the Royal Prince Alfred Hospital Allergy Unit.[7]

Salicylate sensitivity research

The table below shows the percentage of sufferers of certain conditions who reacted adversely to salicylate challenge tests.[8,9]

Eczema	52%
Hives	62–75%
Irritable Bowel Syndrome	69%
Migraines	62%
Behavioural issues (i.e. ADHD, aggression etc. – mostly men)	74%
Systemic (i.e. lethargy, headaches, gut dysbiosis etc. – mostly women)	74%

According to Dr Weston Price, 'Reactions [to salicylates] are caused when arachidonic acid is tripped into the inflammatory chemicals called leukotrienes, causing dilated blood vessels, constricted bronchial passages and mucus production. Salicylates have a cumulative effect in the body and build up over time. Thus some people feel great when they first start a raw vegan diet, only to later develop salicylate intolerance.'[10]

If you have seen countless practitioners and tried dozens of remedies, diets and creams and you still have eczema, you probably have undiagnosed chemical sensitivity. If you are sensitive to salicylates, other eczema treatments will fail until a low-salicylate diet is implemented.

Signs and symptoms of salicylate intolerance and chemical intolerance

Not all salicylate and chemical sensitivity symptoms will be present in one person. Symptoms are varied and they can be mild to severe depending on the individual. Ringing in the ears (tinnitus) is often the first sign to appear in adults with chemical sensitivity.

Symptoms include the following:

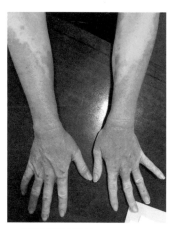

Skin:
eczema/dermatitis/hives/
  rashes
worsening of eczema
sensitive skin
facial flushing
rosacea
psoriasis

Gastrointestinal:
Irritable Bowel Syndrome
diarrhoea
stomach ache
colic/acid reflux
flatulence
leaky gut
bed wetting

Allergy/atopic:
flu-like symptoms
runny nose (nasal drip)
nasal obstruction
sneezing
asthma
perfume intolerance
anaphylactic reactions

Behavioural:
ADHD/ADD
aggressive behaviour
poor attention span
and more …

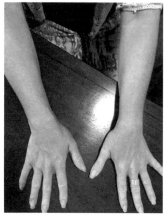

Anna: chronic eczema caused by salicylate intolerance. The photo shows her skin before treatment and after implementing the low-salicylate (FID) program in this book.

Systemic:
ringing in the ears
brain fog
headaches
migraine
fatigue
anxiety
depression
panic attacks

In severe cases, some chemical sensitivities can trigger strong feelings of anger, aggression, suicidal thoughts and physical pain.

These symptoms can be caused by other factors so speak to your doctor if you are concerned.

Case study: my personal account of salicylate intolerance

*My nine-year-old son had occasional **severe abdominal pains** and he missed a lot of school as a result. We saw a couple of gastrointestinal specialists, had X-rays, a stool analysis and allergy testing. Everything showed up clear except for mild **constipation**. We gave him constipation medication and fruit juice but the symptoms persisted. He occasionally became so **anxious** he would hide under the bed and hyperventilate. He often complained of **headaches — all are common signs of salicylate sensitivity**.*

*So after six months of medical tests to rule out more serious causes, I finally tested for salicylate intolerance. My son is a sweet, intelligent child but two years ago he was the child who **could not sit still** in class — he was a wriggler! After a week on the low-salicylate diet I was reading him a book at night and I suddenly noticed he had been completely still for three whole chapters, arms by his side, silent, not reading a second book at the same time. I was alarmed and asked, 'What's wrong?' before remembering he was on the diet. While his school grades were good, his marks improved considerably with no extra study. He no longer suffers from constipation, stomach pains, headaches and anxiety and, best of all, he can handle conflict. For example, if he gets into trouble, instead of having an anxiety attack, getting angry and refusing to go to school, he will complain briefly then calmly let it go. He might even hug me and apologize. My jaw drops each time.*

Many health practitioners do not believe in salicylate sensitivity, so you might have trouble finding a practitioner to support you. But if you never test for salicylate sensitivity you'll never know if it is one of your triggers. Having salicylate sensitivity diagnosed has changed our lives for the better — my son no longer suffers with debilitating pains. My salicylate-sensitive daughter is eczema-free and can now eat a wide range of salicylate-rich foods, thanks to proper diagnosis and treatment.

FAQ

'What causes chemical sensitivity?'

Common triggers include the following:

- nutritional deficiencies
- frequent aspirin consumption
- frequent chemical exposures
- frequent perfume use
- chemicals in cigarettes
- some medications or illicit drugs
- frequent alcohol consumption
- frequent sugar consumption
- fast foods with additives
- crop spraying (on farms)
- illness
- fatty liver
- under-functioning liver (normal in children under 2)
- genetics (occurs in families)
- poor liver detoxification of chemicals

According to research:

- Salicylates are found in many fruits, vegetables, baby teething gel, teas, spices, aspirin, peanuts and most nuts.
- Salicylates are detoxified more slowly in infants than in those with mature liver function.[11]
- Salicylate toxicity can cause eczema, failure to thrive and slowed growth in children.[12,13]

Addressing salicylate sensitivity

Nutrient deficiencies, high chemical exposures and liver dysfunction are the top triggers of salicylate sensitivity, and this book will help you correct these issues. The FID Program can help you diagnose salicylate sensitivity (and other chemical intolerances) and the Eczema Detox Program can help you reverse it.

The programs in this book are designed to improve your health and give your liver a break from high chemical exposures. A rest from chemical overload can do wonders for reducing the itch and clearing up skin inflammation. This enables your body to strengthen so you can consume a wider range of foods, in time. Not everyone will have a chemical intolerance to salicylates — your problem might be amines or tannins or nitrates and MSG. This book, via the FID Program, will help you work out which specific chemicals you are reacting to.

Amine intolerance

Amines are naturally occurring food chemicals formed during protein breakdown and the fermentation process. Very rich sources of amines include probiotics, soy sauce, kefir, miso, tempeh, yeast extracts, cheese, wine, avocado, beer, smoked salmon and chocolate.

How can amines affect eczema sufferers? According to researchers from the Allergy Unit of Sydney's Royal Prince Alfred Hospital, amines trigger hives in 62 per cent of people prone to skin rashes, and trigger eczema in 36 per cent of people prone to eczema.[14] It's important to diagnose amine intolerance before trying fermented foods and other amine-rich products, as they can worsen eczema in some individuals.

Amine intolerance can also trigger irritable bowel symptoms, migraines, behaviour problems, fatigue and a range of systemic symptoms in 62 per cent of people with these symptoms.

The health of your liver is an important part of managing and preventing amine intolerance. Refer 'How to manage amine intolerance' on p. 118–19. If you are unsure if you react to amines, begin with the FID Program in Chapter 9.

Case study: Hana

'I am the mother of a fourteen-month-old girl, Hana, who started to have eczema when she was four months old. Even since she was around seven months, she started to itch and scratch her face and it would bleed to a point of showing raw skin. My prayers were answered after I found The Eczema Diet. *I found out that Hana has sensitivity to salicylates and amines. She reacts to food like broccoli, kale, spinach and probiotics etc. All the food I thought was healthy for her healing. I booked a consultation with Karen and started using the Skin Friend supplement for Hana. It has been four-and-a-half months now and Hana has become a whole new person, a happy baby who doesn't itch her face, a baby who does not need to wear dressings on her face to sleep daily, a normal life for her.'*

KRISTY, UNITED STATES

Glutamate (MSG) intolerance

A study conducted by Loblay and Swain found that 35 per cent of eczema sufferers have adverse reactions to monosodium glutamate, a flavour enhancer that is both natural (i.e. present in tomato and broccoli) and artificial and added to products such as flavoured potato chips and Chinese takeaway food. Dietary MSG can not only worsen eczema symptoms, it may increase the risk of premature wrinkles because it reduces stores of glutathione, an anti-ageing antioxidant enzyme needed for liver detoxification of chemicals.[15]

Common allergy foods for people with eczema include egg, dairy, peanuts, sesame and wheat, and if you are allergic to these foods you must continue to avoid them.

MSG intolerance can trigger or worsen:

» irritable bowel syndrome in 72 per cent of people who are prone to IBS
» migraines in 62 per cent of people prone to migraines
» behavioural problems (ADHD, aggression, anger issues, inattention etc.) in 39 per cent of people with behaviour issues
» systemic (whole body) symptoms in 64 per cent of people with a range of adverse symptoms including skin rashes, fatigue, asthma, mouth ulcers and hay fever.[16]

MSG intolerance varies from person to person and not everyone with eczema will be sensitive to MSG. However, I have found most of my patients react to MSG-rich foods because these foods usually contain salicylates and amines. If you suffer from eczema, it's important to check for MSG/glutamate sensitivity and you can do this via the FID Program in Chapter 8.

Preservatives

Over the last 200 years food manufacturers have introduced highly processed foods containing artificial colours, preservatives, sweeteners and flavour enhancers. Our biological make-up hasn't had enough time to become accustomed to this barrage of artificial additives.[17]

Food preservatives cause a worsening of eczema symptoms in more than 50 per cent of eczema sufferers.[18] It's important to avoid food preservatives in the bid to prevent eczema. Refer to the food additive chart on p. 102.

Sulphites

While dried fruits might be touted as a healthy snack for children, one dried apricot can contain 16 mg of sulphur dioxide, which can cause a worsening of eczema symptoms and a range of adverse reactions such as diarrhoea, unfocused behaviour, hyperactivity, smelly gas and it could trigger an asthma attack in susceptible individuals.[19]

If you've ever experienced facial flushing after drinking a glass of red wine you may be sensitive to sulphites. Sulphites (also known as sulfites), such as sulphur dioxide, are food preservatives which are commonly used to preserve wines, deli meats, grapes, prawns (shrimp), dried fruits and dried vegetables to name a few. Sulphites destroy vitamin B1 and folic acid in foods, so they can be considered an 'anti-nutrient'. So the Eczema Detox is free of sulphite-rich foods.

Nitrates

Nitrates are chemicals used to preserve meats such as bacon, sausages and ham. According to research by Loblay and Swain, eczema sufferers are sensitive to nitrates and nitrate consumption can worsen eczema symptoms in 43 per cent of eczema sufferers.[20]

Nitrates can also damage your liver. According to laboratory studies, the antioxidants quercetin, vitamin C and vitamin E help to reverse the liver damage caused by nitrate consumption.[21,22,23]

Quick search tool

As there are literally hundreds of food additives, if you would like to investigate an additive in a food product, go to www.eczemalife.com and search 'List of food additives to avoid'. Then use the search key on your computer to quickly find the word or number you are looking for. Then see if the additive is listed as 'okay', 'caution' or 'avoid'.

External chemical exposures

It is not only food chemicals that can trigger skin rashes — we are exposed to environmental chemicals every day via pollution, new furnishings, perfumes, chemicals in our skincare products and household cleaners.

Swedish researchers examined children with eczema and their exposure to household concentrations of chemicals emitted from building materials, paints and furniture and found the following:

» Chemicals called PGEs found in bedroom air caused significantly elevated risks of asthma, hay fever and eczema as well as IgE-sensitization (allergic reactions) in preschool age children.[24]

» The researchers concluded 'the risks of PGEs at such low concentrations at home raise concerns for the vulnerability of infants and young children'.[25]

While chemical exposures often cannot be avoided, a few activities to help counteract the damaging effects of chemicals include the following:

1. Ventilate your home: open your windows daily to allow fresh air to enter.
2. Love your liver: it is the chemical processing plant of the body and the best way to counteract daily chemical exposures is to improve the liver's detoxification processes and reduce chemical exposures, where possible. Refer to the Eczema Detox Program in Chapter 9 for more information.

Nutrient deficiencies

The results from a Korean study showed how atopic dermatitis patients had significantly different food preferences and eating habits compared to people with clear skin. The study found that people with eczema had significantly lower intakes of vitamin B1, vitamin B2 and vitamin E than people with clear skin.[26] Furthermore, eczema sufferers did not consume enough calcium and zinc, both of which were remarkably lower than the recommended dietary allowance (RDA, also known as recommended daily intake or RDI) for each nutrient.[27]

Today we have largely forgotten to check for common nutrient deficiencies as a first line treatment for eczema, dermatitis, psoriasis and other skin disorders, possibly because the nutrient deficiency research has been well established for more than 70 years. No one wants to re-establish that deficiencies in biotin, calcium and vitamins B1 and B3 can cause eczema or dermatitis.[28,29] This book contains important supplement information and carefully crafted recipes to reverse nutritional deficiencies and strengthen your skin.

The Itchy Dozen worst foods for eczema

People are often surprised to find the Itchy Dozen includes some of the so-called good foods for eczema. I know the Itchy Dozen contradicts some popular beliefs published in online blogs. However, these foods could be the reason your skin is dry, flaky and incredibly itchy because they are rich in *natural chemicals* such as salicylates.

The Itchy Dozen worst foods for eczema

Food	Research
1. Grapes (sultanas, raisins, wines, grape juice)	Grapes are a 'triple threat' as they are a very rich source of salicylates, amines and MSG.[30] Grapes are also a highly acidic fruit, promoting acid in the body which increases the itch of eczema.
2. Oranges (including orange juice)	Oranges are a strongly acidifying fruit, and a very rich source of salicylates and amines.[31]
3. Kiwi fruit	Kiwi fruit is another strongly acidifying fruit, which is very rich in salicylates and amines.[32]
4. Soy sauce (including tamari and other sushi sauces)	Soy sauce is very rich in amines and MSG (both natural or artificial). According to a Japanese study, consuming chocolate, soy sauce, fermented soybeans, cheese and yoghurt causes a worsening of eczema symptoms. All of the participants in the study had significantly less eczema after they avoided these foods for three months.[33]
5. Tomatoes (tomato sauce/ ketchup, canned tomatoes and tomato juice)	Tomatoes are a 'triple threat' as they are a very rich source of salicylates, amines and natural MSG.[34]
6. Avocado	While avocado is a healthy addition to your diet *when you don't have eczema*, it is one of the richest sources of amines and itch-promoting salicylates.[35]
7. Broccoli	Another 'triple threat' – rich in itch-promoting salicylates, amines and natural MSG.[36]
8. Dried fruits (including apricots, dates, prunes, sultanas etc.)	You could say these are a quadruple threat ... all types of dried fruits contain high levels of itch-promoting salicylates and amines, and some contain the preservative sulphur dioxide and natural MSG, which is why they are flavoursome.[37]

Food	Research
9. Deli meats (sausages, bacon, ham, flavoured meats, devon, salami, etc.)	Deli meats are a rich source of nitrates and are highly acid-forming in the body.[38]
10. Eggs (especially raw egg whites that are hidden in mayonnaise, coleslaw dressings, pancake mix, some dips, egg protein shakes, chocolate mousse and pavlova, etc.)	Between 70–90% of eczema sufferers are allergic or sensitive to eggs. Raw egg whites also contain an anti-nutrient called avidin, which causes a biotin deficiency called 'egg white injury' that can trigger eczema/dermatitis.[39]
11. Chocolate (cocoa, cacao, chocolate milk, coffee, tea)	Chocolate is particularly problematic because of the very high levels of amines and saturated fats, which can cause excess skin dryness, cracking and flaking in people who are sensitive to chemicals. Roasting cocoa and cacao increases the levels of vasoactive amines.[40] Carob is a safe alternative as it's amine- and salicylate-free.
12. Dairy products (cow's milk, yoghurt, cheese, ice-cream, dairy desserts, sheep's and goat's milk)	Researchers found that 89% of eczema sufferers are allergic to dairy products, when the patients were tested via several methods to gain accurate results. They tested children via both the skin prick test and patch test, and included delayed adverse reactions, which are not normally included in regular testing. They found doing only one type of test did not give accurate results.[41] Yoghurt and milk are particularly problematic for people with eczema.

In a nutshell

The main point to take away from this chapter is that eczema can be triggered by chemical intolerance. Your eczema might not be provoked by all of these chemicals, but this book will help you discover your specific triggers so you know what to avoid and how to recover so you can have clear, healthy skin.

Case study: a personal account of chemical intolerance

When baby Clare was brought in to see me she had eczema and was vomiting up to ten times a day and not growing as well as her twin. Clare was placed on a low-salicylate diet and her mother, Jenny, put the other twin on the same diet for convenience. During a return consultation Jenny reported:

'Clare has gone from vomiting up to ten times a day to just once a week. She hasn't had any rashes for at least a fortnight. She stopped vomiting within three to four days after starting the diet and supplements. Her twin sister, Reese, is also a "new" baby girl ... she's gone from a grumpy whinger to a happy little girl in the last few weeks. Reese's personality change happened about two weeks after starting the new diet.'

Chapter 2
About the programs

This book contains three low-salicylate (low-chemical) health programs for eczema and other types of skin inflammation:

- » Skin Supplement Program (Chapter 7)
- » Food Intolerance Diagnosis (FID) Program (Chapter 8)
- » Eczema Detox Program (Chapter 9).

The programs in this book have been designed with the utmost care to ensure every known nutrient is supplied for good health *and improved health*. The two food-based programs contain every food group except for dairy products so the inclusion of a calcium supplement is an essential part of your new routine. The programs include wheat-free wholegrain carbohydrates (only gluten-free if you are gluten intolerant), plus lean protein foods and fish. You may choose to be vegetarian or vegan if you want to, but this is not a requirement of the detox. The programs are low in sugar and caffeine-free.

The goal is to temporarily restrict the diet — and therefore get well — then expand the diet. How long this takes varies from person to person, so be patient as it can take time. It helps immensely if your family members are 'on board' and follow the program with you, at least part of the time. You can also do the programs on your own — you are the one who will benefit the most.

While more than 89 per cent of people have success on these diets and the Skin Supplement Program, if you still have eczema after about three months on the FID Program, you can do additional investigative work to uncover *undiagnosed food intolerance* which could be preventing your skin from completely clearing up. See Chapter 12, 'FAQs and problem solving'.

The programs in this book are for people with the following health problems:

- » allergies
- » asteatotic eczema (eczema craquelé)
- » atopic dermatitis (dermatitis)
- » Candida (*Candida albicans*)
- » contact dermatitis
- » cradle cap
- » dandruff
- » discoid eczema (nummular eczema)
- » dyshidrotic eczema (pompholyx eczema)
- » eczema, atopic eczema (all types)
- » eczema herpeticum
- » gravitational eczema (varicose eczema, stasis eczema)
- » ichthyosis vulgaris (scaly, dry skin)
- » keratosis pilaris
- » topical steroid withdrawal
- » red skin syndrome
- » hidradenitis suppurativa
- » psoriasis
- » seborrheic dermatitis
- » food sensitivities
- » chemical sensitivities
- » salicylate sensitivity
- » amine sensitivity
- » glutamate/MSG sensitivity
- » sulphite sensitivity
- » increased intestinal permeability (leaky gut)
- » and more

Note: it's important to avoid self-diagnosing your skin condition as there are many different types of skin abnormalities and some may require medical attention. If you haven't had a doctor diagnose your skin condition, see your GP before starting the Eczema Detox. You can then choose the program from the book best suited for your needs.

Handy cooking appliances

I recommend the following cooking appliances as they make the programs enjoyable and easy to follow:

- · a high-powered blender, rather than a regular blender (there are plenty of cheap ones; anything like a NutriBullet will do)
- · a non-stick waffle maker (they are super cheap and new is better as you will use less oil)
- · a juicing machine (ideally a slow/cold pressed juicer but any type will do).

Chapter 3
Before you begin: do this now

Here are some tips to help you before starting one of the programs:

- » Before beginning your new eczema program, eat and enjoy your favourite meals.
- » Use the foods currently in your refrigerator but do not restock them once they run out. Then, once you've decided which program is right for you, do a grocery shop using the Eczema Detox food shopping list (pp. 92–3) or the FID Program food shopping list (p. 78) before you begin.
- » If you currently drink tea or coffee daily, or frequently consume other caffeinated products including green tea, chai tea, chocolate, cacao, soft drinks (sodas) or energy drinks, then follow 'Caffeine/sugar withdrawal week' below before beginning your chosen program.
- » If you love sugary foods also follow the 'Caffeine/sugar withdrawal week' information below before beginning your chosen program.
- » If you have a child with eczema, gradually cut down on their sugar intake. If you buy sweets and packaged food, start looking at the labels and find the additive-free versions (see 'Eczema-friendly party treats' on p. 79 for tips).
- » Buy your new skin care products or 100 per cent cotton sheets (or whatever eczema prop you need) before beginning this diet so you can test the diet separately. Some people do everything at the same time and then don't know what has helped their skin. Be like a scientist conducting an experiment and test one thing at a time.

Caffeine/sugar withdrawal week

Caffeine and sugar are highly addictive, so when you stop consuming them your body can experience withdrawal symptoms, similar to a drug addict's reaction when abstaining from their drug of choice.

Caffeine and sugar withdrawal symptoms include:

» itchy skin	» aches and pains	» fatigue
» cravings	» headaches	» constipation
» bingeing	» body tremors	» depression
» anxiety	» fuzzy head	» nausea
» moodiness	» sleepiness	» flu-like symptoms

Don't worry — it will pass, you'll feel much better afterwards, and your skin will thank you!

Sources of caffeine include:

- » coffee
- » black tea
- » English breakfast tea
- » Earl Grey tea
- » green tea
- » chai tea
- » iced tea
- » cola soft drinks (sodas)
- » non-cola soft drinks (sodas)

- » energy drinks
- » chocolate
- » hot chocolate
- » cacao
- » cocoa beans
- » kola nuts (herbal)
- » guarana berries
- » yerba mate
- » mate tea
- » matcha (green tea powder)

- » weight loss pills
- » pain relievers
- » breath fresheners
- » ice-cream
- » some snack foods
- » some multivitamin supplements
- » some herbal supplements

Why tea is bad for your skin

There are hundreds of blogs touting the virtues of caffeine-rich teas such as matcha, chai and green tea. However in reality, if you have eczema then most teas are probably hurting your skin due to the high content of itch-promoting chemicals. From my personal experience, giving up my beloved cup of chai tea was very hard to do. I had to stop drinking tea and eating chocolate as they caused body aches and my skin looked dry and red. Now I am 100 per cent caffeine-free and my health has never been better. I no longer wake up tired and needing a caffeine fix, my energy levels are steady and good, I have no more body aches, no more red skin around my mouth, no more stained teeth, and my nails are a hundred times stronger.

The following scientific research helped me to quit the caffeine.

Teas block DAO activity (this is important!)

In the body, diamine oxidase (DAO) is the main enzyme that breaks down histamine. Monoaminoxidase (MAO) also plays a role in histamine breakdown. According to German researchers, MAO and DAO activity are significantly decreased in patients with atopic eczema, compared with people without eczema.[1]

According to research published in the *American Journal of Clinical Nutrition*, DAO activity can be blocked by the consumption of tea, alcohol, food additives, nicotine and heavy metals such as mercury.[2] So they can prevent your body's natural antihistamine mechanisms from working properly. The result is atopic skin inflammation, hay fever and increased allergic responses.

Avoid the following, which contain DAO blockers:

- » alcohol
- » black tea
- » green tea
- » mate tea
- » energy drinks
- » all forms of caffeine
- » nicotine
- » food additives
- » mercury

FAQ

'Do I need to do the caffeine/sugar withdrawal week or can I begin the Eczema Detox/FID Program immediately?'

Be patient and do them separately or it will be confusing. For example, let's say you begin the FID Program and on the same day you stop consuming caffeine and sugar. The FID Program elimination period is for only two weeks but for that whole two weeks you experience terrible caffeine withdrawal symptoms. Now you wonder if the diet is the problem. You don't attribute your symptoms to caffeine/ sugar withdrawal and you become disheartened. Once your caffeine withdrawal symptoms have subsided you now need to redo the FID Program.

If you are following the Eczema Detox Program I also suggest doing the caffeine withdrawal week separately so you can see the untainted results of the diet.

Caffeine/sugar withdrawal tips

Withdrawing from caffeine addiction is difficult and can take time. However, once you have successfully withdrawn you should have newfound energy. Here are some tips to help you feel good during the withdrawal week:

- » Drink plenty of filtered water (adults should have 1.5 to 3 litres/3 to 6 pints per day)
- » Rest and relax.
- » Exercise to restore hormone balance.
- » Take B vitamins to boost your energy (see Chapter 7, 'Skin Supplement Program').

Switch to decaf (if you're desperate)

A cup of coffee contains around 65 mg of caffeine while decaf coffee contains only 3 mg. So it can be useful to avoid all caffeine-rich products on the list and switch to decaf coffee so you are consuming a much smaller dose of caffeine. This can help to reduce withdrawal symptoms. Note that decaf coffee is low in salicylates (more on this shortly), so it is allowed in moderation while following the diet, but some people adversely react to decaf. You can also try Carob Tea as a chocolate substitute (see p. 126). Refer to the health benefits of carob on p. 46.

People with tannin sensitivity

A small number of eczema sufferers are tannin intolerant so be aware that decaf coffee, carob and pears contain tannins. If you react to these ingredients, suspect tannin intolerance. A sign of mild tannin/chemical intolerance is ringing in the ears (tinnitus) after consuming these substances.

Non-aspirin pain medications

Avoid aspirin, unless medically prescribed, as it is very rich in salicylates and as a result it can worsen skin inflammation. Colour-free paracetamol or acetaminophen (the US equivalent) are safer options if used as directed for a short period of time. People on medications should seek advice from their doctor regarding painkillers. Ideally, avoid using painkillers if you have eczema.

Information for people with leaky gut

Many people associate eczema with 'leaky gut' (the official term is 'increased intestinal permeability'). These are the eczema sufferers who have gut symptoms such as the following (all symptoms will not be present in everyone, but you may have several):

- » constipation
- » diarrhoea
- » excessive gas
- » abdominal pains
- » excessive bloating (not regular bloating)
- » undigested food in stools
- » discoloured stools
- » abdominal pain after eating
- » gluten intolerance
- » Irritable Bowel Syndrome
- » nutritional deficiencies

If this sounds like you, then do a brief gut-healing regime by taking a pure glutamine supplement *for ten days*. Glutamine is an amino acid from protein which heals the cells in your gut lining. So if needed, take glutamine along with weaning yourself off caffeine and sugar before beginning one of the programs in this book.

I repeat, glutamine is not to be taken indefinitely, only for ten days. It's a wonderful nutrient but it's not for everyone. This routine is deliberately brief as glutamine contains glutamates (similar to MSG), which some eczema sufferers adversely react to. If you know you are sensitive to MSG/glutamates do not take glutamine. Most people are unaware if they react to glutamates but this book will help you work it out. Note the diet in this book is also designed to heal your gut lining — glutamine can speed this up for those who have abdominal pains and are not sensitive to glutamates.

Glutamine dosages

· Adults: 10–20 g per day taken in divided doses (i.e. 5 g taken 2–4 times daily)
· Children (over age 1): 500 mg (0.5 g) to 3 g per day taken in divided doses (i.e. older children can have 1 g taken 3 times daily). The lowest dose is for younger children.

Instructions: Mix the powdered glutamine into water, and take before meals on an empty stomach or in between meals (not with food or other supplements, and avoid vitamin A glutamine mixes). Begin on a lower dose for the first 4 days. Buy a pure powder form, not capsules as you may not digest them properly.

Note: glutamine is not suitable for pregnant or breastfeeding women.

Why healthy foods can be unhealthy for eczema

Go to eczemalife.com and search for 'Why healthy foods can be unhealthy for eczema'. This article covers the imbalances in the two types of 'helper' cells in the immune system — Th1 and Th2 — seen in a wide range of skin disorders, including eczema. Find out what popular ingredients worsen Th2-dominated conditions such as eczema — the list will surprise you. It also covers ingredients to balance your immune system.

Chapter 4

Choose your program

After fifteen years working with skin disorder patients, I have found three programs that are most helpful: the Skin Supplement Program, the Eczema Detox Program and the Food Intolerance Diagnosis (FID) Program.

So which program is right for you?

Level 1: Skin Supplement Program

This program is ideal for people with *mild* skin rashes and recent eczema (i.e. you've had eczema for a month, not years). It's also suitable for people who cannot follow a diet program due to frequent travel. Or, if you are a teenager at boarding school you might like to begin with this program. If you need to change programs to speed up your results, you can try the FID program when you are at home during the holidays. For more information about the Skin Supplement Program see Chapter 7.

At a glance: the Skin Supplement Program

The Skin Supplement Program is best suited for	Not suitable for	Recommendations
· People with nutritional deficiencies · Mild eczema or dermatitis · Mild skin inflammation · Newly diagnosed skin inflammation · Skin inflammation for less than 6 months · Have not used topical steroids for more than three months (or not frequently) · Current topical steroid use and successfully managing eczema · People who travel frequently · Allergies and intolerances that have been diagnosed · Acne	· Babies under age 1 (see baby program on p. 105) · Severe eczema · Lifelong eczema · Topical steroid withdrawal (recently stopped steroid treatments) – these conditions are better suited to the other two programs	Duration: Treatment can be ongoing. If your symptoms persist past 12 weeks, progress to the other two programs in this book. See Chapter 7 for the Skin Supplement Program and read the information in this book to see if you need further help.

Level 2: The Eczema Detox Program

This program relies on fresh vegetable juices, supplements and healthy recipes to boost the health of the liver, balance the immune system (reduce Th2) and strengthen the health of the whole body. It's ideal for people with mild to moderate eczema and mild food intolerances. The Eczema Detox Program contains a wider variety of foods than the Food Intolerance Diagnosis (FID) Program. It is a healthy, low- to medium-salicylate detox program and it includes a few amine-containing foods for variety. For more information about the Eczema Detox Program see Chapter 9.

Note: if you have undiagnosed allergies or severe chemical intolerances then you may need the FID Program.

At a glance: the Eczema Detox Program

The Eczema Detox Program is best suited for	Not suitable for	Recommendations
· People in good health · People with nutritional deficiencies · People who know their trigger/allergy foods · People who feel good on alkalizing diets (for acid–alkaline balance) · Mild, moderate to severe eczema and dermatitis · All types of skin rashes · Those currently using topical steroids or recently stopped · Those with diagnosed allergies and intolerances · People with topical steroid withdrawal/red skin syndrome · Acne	· Babies under age 1 (see Baby program on p. 105) · Those with multiple chemical sensitivities · People who are highly salicylate intolerant · Those with low stomach acid and who do better on acidic diets · If you are pregnant, breastfeeding or taking medications consult with your doctor before changing your diet	Duration: As long as necessary. If your symptoms persist past 12 weeks then try the FID Program as you may have undiagnosed food intolerances. See Chapter 9 for the Eczema Detox Program and read the information in this book to see if you need further help.

Level 3: Food Intolerance Diagnosis (FID) Program

The Food Intolerance Diagnosis Program (or FID Program for short) is a diagnostic program for adults and children with moderate, severe or stubborn eczema, psoriasis and other skin rashes. It's for people who have tried everything and 'nothing has helped'. It's also ideal for people who have followed my previous book, *The Eczema Diet*, and need more help.

- » If you don't know what your trigger foods are, this program is for you.
- » If you avoid your allergy foods and you still have painful skin inflammation that is driving you mad and you want quick answers, this program is for you.
- » People who have completed the FID Program can often progress to the Eczema Detox Program as their skin improves.

I usually prescribe the FID Program to my patients who have had lifelong eczema, or widespread eczema, or signs of chemical sensitivities and they want fast relief. It is the strictest of the three regimes and you need to spend time preparing food and cooking on this program. For more information about the FID Program see Chapter 8.

At a glance: the FID Program

The FID Program is best suited for	Not suitable for	Recommendations
· People with chemical sensitivities or salicylate intolerance · People who often feel tired and unwell · People who know their allergy foods but are unsure about intolerances · Mild, moderate to severe eczema and dermatitis · All types of skin rashes · Those currently using topical steroids · People with TSW/red skin syndrome · People with controlled autoimmune diseases (check with your GP first)	· Babies under age 1 (it is fine to follow this program with medical supervision) · People who are frail	Duration: 2 weeks on the restricted diet, then 4+ weeks testing foods. If you have severe or lifelong eczema it can be longer. See Chapter 8 for the FID Program.

FAQs

'Can I be vegan while following your programs?'

If you are vegan or vegetarian, the Eczema Detox and FID programs can be suitable for you as there are many vegan and vegetarian options within the recipes. Ensure you are taking supplements to fill nutritional gaps, such as iron, B12 and vegan omega-3, and ensure you are eating vegetarian protein foods daily including lentils, beans and tofu if you are not sensitive to soy (see vegan supplement information on p 57). Pea protein powder (no flavouring or other ingredients) is also an option to increase your protein intake.

'I like to eat paleo; is there an option to do this within the book?'

Yes and no. If you prefer eating paleo there are some paleo-style recipes within this book. You can limit your carbohydrate intake on the Eczema Detox or FID programs *if you are sensitive to grains* (8 per cent of eczema sufferers are sensitive to grains and starch – so this number is quite small). If you are *not* sensitive to grains it's best to stick within the recipe guidelines for best results (plus avoid your trigger foods). Note that excessive saturated fat from animal sources can worsen eczema, so while on this program eat lean meats with the fat removed – this is essential. Adding alkaline carbohydrate-rich vegetables such as beetroot (beets) and sweet potato to your detox regime (instead of grains) is an option.

If you are sensitive to grains (i.e. you suspect your skin worsens when you eat rice and bread etc.) please continue to avoid your trigger foods. Of the hundreds of eczema patients I see each year, I've had only one patient who was sensitive to all grains and whenever he tried to incorporate grains such as rice back into his diet his eczema flared up. He now happily avoids all grains and that works for his particular case. Some eczema cases are unique and it's important to acknowledge that. For others, however, this style of eating could prevent eczema from clearing up.

Keep in mind the paleo, GAPS and autoimmune paleo programs are all high in salicylates, histamines/amines and saturated fats, so they cannot be used in conjunction with the programs in this book. If you wish to follow them please do – try them for as long as desired, then if you need further help, stop your routine and then start the Eczema Detox. Look at changing your diet to a low-chemical detox as 'detective work' to see if this style of eating clears up your skin.

'I like to eat fish and seafood, but not meat. Can the programs in your book be pescatarian?'

Yes, you can eat fish and you do not have to eat meat. Note that store-bought prawns usually contain preservatives so they are not part of the program, and some other types of seafood might not be suitable due to high mercury levels. Fresh (not frozen) small white fish such as flathead and hake are usually best. You can also enjoy fresh salmon if you are following the Eczema Detox Program (not the

FID Program for the first three weeks). Note some people are sensitive to seafood and they are unaware of this — if you are unsure you are sensitive to fish, do the FID Program (Chapter 8) and test fish in week 4.

Important allergy note

The Eczema Detox and FID programs are designed to help you identify undiagnosed allergies and intolerances, so you can avoid these foods and heal your skin inflammation. While it is important to strictly follow the programs, there are exceptions:

Know your lingo

Atopic: describes an allergy-prone individual and includes eczema, asthma and hay fever.

Dermatitis: any generalized inflammation of the skin.

Eczema: derived from a Greek word meaning 'to boil out'.

» If you are allergic to an ingredient continue to avoid that ingredient, i.e. if a recipe has that ingredient, use a substitute from the shopping list or choose a different recipe.

» If you have known food intolerances continue to avoid these foods for the time being. If you do not have anaphylaxis, you might like to test the foods again in a few months' time to see if you are still sensitive. Sometimes people have to avoid their trigger foods long term, but often it is possible to grow out of intolerances once your health has been restored.

» If you are taking prescription medications for any disease keep taking your prescribed medications if needed.

Skin disorders, causes and treatments

Here is a brief table of skin disorders, causes and treatments. For food sources and dosages of supplements mentioned below, refer to Chapter 7 on the Skin Supplement Program. To view this table with images of the skin disorders, go to www.eczemalife.com and search 'Skin disorders'.

Skin disorder	Causes/triggers	Treatments
Asteatotic eczema (eczema craquelé) – like crazy paving	Ageing (usually occurs over age 60), nutritional deficiencies, topical steroid use (skin disorder appears when topical steroids discontinued), also triggered by soaps and detergents.	Check for nutritional deficiencies and food chemical intolerances (see FID Program, Chapter 8). Check protein intake (may need plain unflavoured pea protein powder); supplements (see 'Eczema' p. 32); avoid harsh soaps and detergents, use 24-hour Rescue Balm or another thick ointment to suit the individual. If you are taking medications, see supplement contraindications in the Skin Supplement Program chapter.
Atopic dermatitis (Chronic and allergy-prone, more severe than other rashes)	Caused by poor diet, poor digestion, stress, sensitivity to salicylates, amines, glutamates (MSG), environmental allergies, low calcium levels in the skin.	Identify nutritional deficiencies, follow FID Program to diagnose if chemical intolerances are involved, recommend allergy testing. Supplement with EPA (omega-3 from algae, or fish oils if no allergy), calcium carbonate to reduce acidity in the body and magnesium, biotin, vitamins B1, B2, B3, B6, zinc, and vitamin C (Skin Friend AM). Avoid vitamin A (retinol forms).
Contact dermatitis	Direct contact with irritants (e.g. latex, nickel, cheap jewellery, hairdressing chemicals), stress, sensitivity to soaps and detergents, nutritional deficiencies.	Reduce stress and increase rest; avoid contact irritants; supplement with molybdenum, magnesium, zinc, B vitamins and calcium (Skin Friend AM). Contraindicated: Avoid vitamin A (retinol forms; beta-carotene is fine) and avoid high-dose vitamin B5 (under 10 mg is fine or RDI) as they worsen dry skin flaking.

Skin disorder	Causes/triggers	Treatments
Cradle cap – yellow crusts on the scalps of babies under age 2	Malabsorption of fats, under-functioning liver (normal for babies under age 2).	Gentle shampoo to wash scalp; use jojoba oil and a fine-toothed comb to gently comb the crusts off. Low-chemical diet (FID Program) is gentle on the liver.
Dermatitis herpetiformis – watery, itchy blisters	Associated with gluten intolerance, Coeliac disease and leaky gut (increased intestinal permeability) .	Take a pure powder glutamine supplement to heal the gut lining (see p. 25 for dosages) and follow the FID Program to diagnose food intolerances (gluten-free version).
Eczema (atopic eczema) – must be itchy to be eczema Discoid eczema (nummular eczema) – coin shaped Dyshidrotic eczema Pompholyx eczema – blisters Gravitational eczema (varicose eczema, stasis eczema)	Babies: genetics and under-functioning liver – results in difficulty detoxifying chemicals (normal for under age 2)[1] Other: nutritional deficiencies, poor detoxification of chemicals, allergies, chemical sensitivities, stress, environmental triggers, those with eczema tend to have increased acid in the body; 34% of children with eczema have fatty liver.[2]	Follow FID Program to diagnose chemical intolerances (i.e. salicylate, MSG, amine and sulphite sensitivity).[3] Supplement with *low dose* B vitamins, biotin, magnesium and zinc (Skin Friend AM), omega-3 (from organic flaxseed oil and fish oil if you are not sensitive to seafood). Calcium carbonate is a salicylate sensitivity remedy (not calcium citrate, as it has an acid attached so it's not alkaline enough). Quality protein in the diet (trim fat off meats), exercise, reduce stress. Contraindicated: avoid vitamin A (retinol forms; beta-carotene is fine) and high vitamin B5 dosages as they cause severe dry skin flaking.
Eczema herpeticum – blistery rash	Topical steroid use (abuse); wet wraps with steroid creams then exposure to infection (i.e. herpes virus).	Zinc and high dose lysine, plus check for nutritional deficiencies; antiviral medications may be prescribed by your doctor; nutritional support is important. See 'Eczema', above.

Skin disorder	Causes/triggers	Treatments
Hidradenitis suppurativa (acne inversa) – inflammatory follicular skin disease	Looks like red, inflamed tunnels in the skin of armpits, groin and upper thighs. Can be caused by metabolic syndrome, obesity, hormones or self-medication by smoking, drinking alcohol, ingesting chemicals or drugs.	Quit smoking program, management of stress, self-nurturing and lifestyle changes are often required. Avoid chemicals such as deodorants, soft drinks/sodas, smoking, fast foods etc. Follow low-chemical detox or FID Program to identify your triggers. Triggers may include sugar, caffeine, dairy, alcohol, nightshades (tobacco, cayenne, paprika, tomato, eggplant/aubergine, potatoes, capsicum/bell peppers, tomatillos and goji berries/wolfberries). Supplement with Skin Friend AM (zinc, vitamin C, biotin, B6, B3, magnesium and calcium) and quality non-dairy pea protein powder (no flavourings).
Ichthyosis vulgaris (scaly, dry skin)	Genetic, possibly from nutritional deficiencies.	Omega-3, zinc, calcium; check chemical sensitivities and deficiencies.
Keratosis pilaris – blocked hair follicles	Vitamin A and EFA (omega-3) deficiencies.	Supplement with natural beta-carotene and omega-3; check for deficiencies.
Perioral dermatitis – around mouth	Topical steroid use, food allergies and food intolerances, sodium lauryl sulfate, parrafin, toothpastes, cosmetics, nutrient deficiencies, stress.	Change skin care and ensure toothpaste is free of sodium lauryl sulfate and other sulfates; take zinc, vitamin B2, B5, B6, folate (levomefolate) and natural beta-carotene. Check for nutrient deficiencies (p. 15).
Psoriasis – silvery plaques, autoimmune	Healthy skin cells turn over every ~28 days but with psoriasis skin cells turn over every 3–4 days (the body is trying to eliminate toxins through the skin). Commonly seen in smokers, triggered by stress and high chemical exposures such as nicotine, pesticides, salicylates.	Follow the Eczema Detox Program or FID Program to diagnose chemical intolerances (check tannins, salicylates, amines, nightshades, etc.). Check for nutrient deficiencies. Take low-chemical liver detoxification nutrients: amino acids, low dose B vitamins, biotin, zinc, calcium, vitamin C (such as Skin Friend AM). Don't place an extra burden on the liver: avoid irritants such as smoking and alcohol, and limit stress (if severe psoriasis, a change in lifestyle).

Skin disorder	Causes/triggers	Treatments
Rosacea	Triggered by amine sensitivity, histamines, sulphites in wines, sedentary lifestyle, poor blood supply to the skin (in rosacea the blood vessels widen to allow 'sluggish' blood quicker access to the skin). May become permanent if not treated.	Avoid amines/histamines as they trigger flushing symptoms, check for salicylate and sulphite sensitivity. Follow FID Program to identify triggers. Exercise daily — it is the best remedy for rosacea as it brings a fresh supply of nutrient-rich blood to the skin and helps restore blood vessel tone/health. Initially, exercise can make it feel worse so ease into it. Use a mini trampoline and keep a fan and ice pack handy.
Seborrheic dermatitis — on scalp and face	Greasy yellowish flakes and itching where oil (sebaceous) glands appear. May begin as dandruff. *Pityrosporum ovale* (a yeast, also known as *Malassezia furfur*) is on the skin of people with seborrheic dermatitis; antibiotic overuse can trigger it.	Check for nutritional deficiencies. Take biotin, reduce sugar intake, gentle scalp treatments (if you are not too sensitive add 1 or 2 teaspoons of quality apple cider vinegar to shampoo). Follow Eczema Detox Program or use FID Program to diagnose chemical intolerances.
Scleroderma — autoimmune	'Fibrous degeneration of connective tissue caused by excessive acidity in the body'.[4]	Follow FID Program: diagnose food/chemical intolerances (also check for tannin intolerance). Avoid your trigger foods once diagnosed. Eat more alkalizing foods (low-chemical ones such as mung bean sprouts, beetroot/beets); zinc gluconate.[5] Low dose B vitamins (avoid high doses above 5 mg as B vitamins are acidic). Check for deficiencies such as vitamin D.

Skin disorder	Causes/triggers	Treatments
Red skin syndrome (RSS) (TSW, mimics rosacea)	Topical steroid withdrawal (TSW)	Check for nutritional deficiencies (hair loss, cracked corners of mouth, insomnia, cracked lips etc.). Avoid/limit salicylates as they increase nitric oxide which worsens skin redness. Follow Eczema Detox or FID programs to identify chemical intolerances. TSW can cause fatty liver, so check for fatty liver (ultrasound if indicated). See 'Eczema' and 'Rosacea' in this table for supplement and exercise advice.
Vitiligo – depigmented skin	Highest incidence occurs in India, and possibly linked to high phenol/tannin content of Indian foods.[6] Tannins chelate metal ions (causing mineral deficiencies) and elevate levels of interleukin-1α (IL-1α) as seen in vitiligo.	Follow the FID Program – plus low tannins – to diagnose if tannins and chemical intolerance are involved. Identify mineral/nutrient deficiencies; avoid tannin-rich foods (i.e. teas, coffee, green tea, wine, beer, chocolate, cacao, carob, apples, pears, bananas, berries, rhubarb, spices, nuts, avocados, vanilla, dates, cinnamon, grapes, pomegranates, oranges, etc).

If you are taking medications, or are pregnant or breastfeeding check with your doctor before taking supplements or changing your diet.

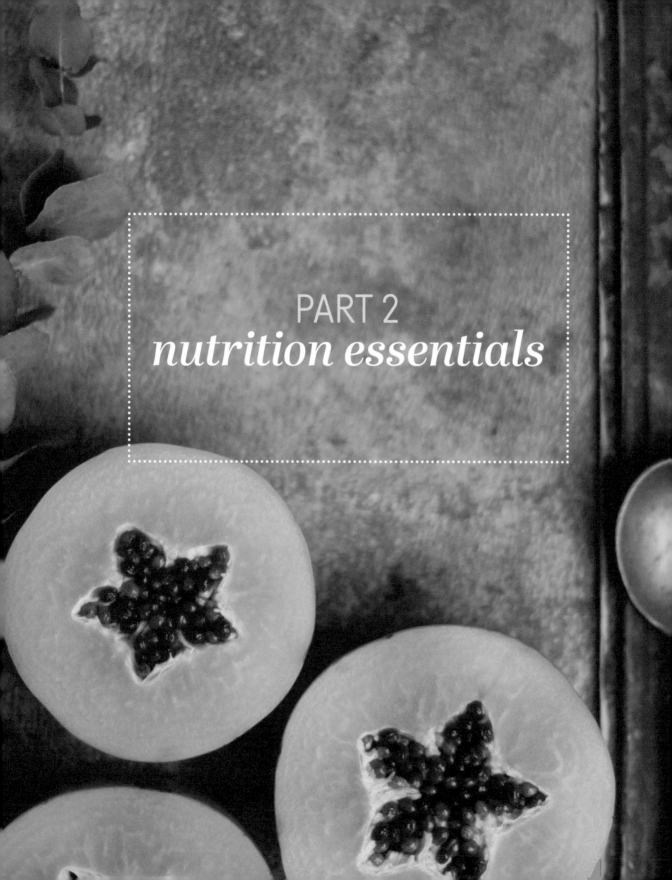

PART 2
nutrition essentials

Chapter 5
Top 12 foods for eliminating eczema

While salicylate-rich foods, such as avocado, tomato, citrus fruits and kiwi fruit can worsen skin rashes, there are a range of foods that are beneficial for preventing and reducing skin inflammation. This chapter features the top 12.

1. Mung bean sprouts

Mung bean sprouts are like little alkalizing 'bombs' when added to your meals as they are one of the few *strongly* alkalizing foods available. They contain magnesium, vitamin K, folate, potassium and vitamin C and they are salicylate-free. Sprouting your own mung beans is easy and the sprouting recipe is on p. 169.

Storage and serving tips

- » Store mung bean sprouts in the refrigerator — they will last about a week but discard them if they turn brown.
- » Always rinse them in water before serving.
- » Add mung bean sprouts to salads and savoury dishes. They also make a healthy addition to children's snacks (kids might prefer them served without the green shells).

Recipes with mung bean sprouts include Mung Bean Sprout Pancakes (p. 168) and Papaya Rice Paper Rolls (p. 208).

Know your sprouts

Mung bean sprouts are the little oval-shaped sprouts with green ends, not the long white sprouts which are often called bean sprouts in the United States. Refer to the 'Specialty ingredients' image on p. 51.

---

2. Flaxseed oil

Flaxseeds, also known as linseeds, are small brown seeds best known for their rich content of anti-inflammatory omega-3 oils. The seeds are a source of phytochemicals including a moderate amount of salicylates and amines, plus silica, mucilage, oleic acid, protein, vitamin E and dietary fibre for gastrointestinal and liver health.

Flaxseed oil is more refined than whole flaxseeds so it contains fewer salicylates and amines and more of the beneficial oils, including 57 per cent omega-3 essential fatty acids. So I suggest beginning with a small bottle of organic flaxseed oil and using it in smoothies (or buy capsules). Then if you find the oil beneficial (and don't react to the small amount of phytochemicals) you can progress to using the whole flaxseeds — these are great sprinkled onto breakfast cereals.

Know your lingo: what is 'alkalizing'?

Throughout this book you will see the word *alkalizing* — this is the term used to describe if a food has alkalizing properties, as opposed to *acidifying* foods such as meats and grains. Eczema is an overly acidic condition where your body produces excess arachidonic acid, which is part of the inflammation process. Consuming alkalizing foods can help to balance your body's acid–alkaline pH when it is overly acidic. Modern western diets can cause low-grade metabolic acidosis, which can worsen eczema. The food shopping list in this chapter includes some powerful alkalizing foods that are also low in chemicals.

Flaxseed oil benefits (when consumed)

» Remedy for dry skin.
» Prevents/reduces dry eyes.
» May prevent constipation.
» Reduces the risk of cancer.
» Promotes healthy hair and nails.
» Promotes healthy skin.
» May reduce cholesterol levels.
» Increases satiety when taken before or with foods.
» Plays a role in burning body fat.
» May reduce menopause symptoms.
» May reduce feelings of anxiety and depression.
» May improve gum/dental health.
» May help mild arthritic pain.

Storage and serving tips

- » Choose quality organic flaxseed oil (which is non-GMO).
- » Omega-3 is highly unstable so it's easily damaged by heat, so do not use flaxseed oil in cooking and keep the bottle in the refrigerator.
- » Don't purchase flaxseed oil that has not been refrigerated in the shop. Flaxseed oil should be used within five weeks of opening or choose capsules, as the encapsulated oils are less likely to go rancid and will last longer.

Daily amount

Below is a guide to the recommended daily amounts of flaxseeds/linseeds.

- » Children aged 1–4: ½–1 teaspoon ground flaxseeds daily* (or ¼ teaspoon flaxseed oil).
- » Older children: 1–2 teaspoons daily* (or ½ teaspoon flaxseed oil).
- » Adults: 2–4 teaspoons daily* (or ½–3 teaspoons flaxseed oil).

*Drink plenty of water when eating flaxseeds as the fibre absorbs about five times the seeds' weight.

Place whole flaxseeds into a coffee or seed grinder and grind them to a fine powder. Grind linseeds weekly to ensure freshness and store them in a sealed glass container in the refrigerator.

3. Red cabbage

Cabbage is another alkalizing vegetable and a member of the mighty brassica family. It's rich in vitamin C, folate and anti-cancer indoles. But it's worth swapping from white cabbage to the red variety as red cabbage has double the amount of dietary fibre compared to regular cabbage and it contains protective purple pigments. These pigments are caused by a group of antioxidants called anthocyanins (a type of tannin), which are powerful flavonoids that have a skin-protective effect against UV sunlight when consumed frequently. Anthocyanins help to protect blood vessels from oxidative damage, and their anti-inflammatory properties activate the production of collagen for healthy skin.

Storage and serving tips

- » Store cabbage in the refrigerator, wrapped in a paper towel and in a sealed plastic bag or container.

» While you can eat raw cabbage, it is recommended to steam or stir-fry cabbage as cooking deactivates the goitrogens (which can affect the thyroid, especially if you have thyroid problems).

Eat cabbage twice a week to gain the health benefits. Recipes include Steamed Fish Parcels with Mashed Potato (p. 172), Pink Pear Jam (p. 137) and Pumpkin and Snow Pea Bowl (p. 197).

4. Spring onions (scallions, shallots)

Spring onions, also referred to as scallions and shallots, are part of the onion family and, like the onion, spring onions contain histamine-lowering, anti-inflammatory quercetin. They have a straight green stem, with no bulb (see the photo 'Specialty ingredients' on p. 51). Like garlic (but in lower concentrations) spring onions possess antioxidant flavonoids that convert to allicin when cut or crushed. Lab experiments show that allicin helps liver cells to reduce cholesterol and has antibacterial, antiviral and antifungal properties, so it's a beneficial ingredient for preventing *Candida albicans* infestation.

Spring onions contain folate, vitamin C, beta-carotene and lutein and are one of the richest sources of vitamin K, which is vital for healthy skin. Just 50 g of raw spring onions provides 103 mcg of vitamin K, nearly double the daily adequate intake for adults.

Storage and serving tips

» Cut the spring onions (shallots, scallions) in half and store them in a sealed container with a few paper towels to absorb excess moisture.
» Spring onions will last one to two weeks in the refrigerator if bought fresh and stored correctly.
» They can be served raw or lightly fried.

Recipes include Lentil Vegie Soup (p. 164); and Alkaline Bomb Salad (p. 153).

Note: spring onions are often mistaken for other types of onions, so refer to the 'Specialty ingredients' image (p. 51) to see what spring onions look like.

5. Fish

Fish is a great source of protein, vitamin D, iodine and anti-inflammatory omega-3. High fish intake during pregnancy is associated with a decreased risk of eczema. Two to three servings of fish each week are beneficial for elevating mood and increasing the health of the brain, skin and heart. Good sources of omega-3, EPA and DHA (these are the converted omega-3 fatty acids) include trout, salmon, sardines, herring and fish oil supplements. Other minor sources of EPA and DHA include low-fat seafood such as carp, pike, haddock and squid.

It's important to favour eczema-safe fish that is low in mercury. The following fish and seafoods are low in mercury, as is the case with all small-sized fish (if in doubt ask your local fishmonger). The general rule is: the higher up the food chain and the bigger the fish (e.g. shark/flake), the more mercury it may contain.

Tip: if you are allergic or sensitive to seafood, avoid fish. If you find your skin improves when you eat fish, you can eat the following fresh fish once or twice a week.

If you are following the low-chemical FID Program, eat:

» flathead
» hake
» flounder
» dory (small fillets)
» bream
» herring

If you are *not* sensitive to amines or salicylates (and not following the FID Program) you can also eat:

» trout and rainbow trout (contain high levels of amines)
» sardines (contain high amines)
» salmon (contains high amines)

Fish to avoid

The following fish contain high levels of mercury and should be avoided. Health authorities recommend if you eat a serving of mercury-rich fish you should then avoid eating all seafood for at least two weeks afterwards, to allow time for your mercury levels to reduce.

Avoid these high-mercury fish:

» flake/shark (often used for fish and chips)
» large snapper
» swordfish
» marlin
» king mackerel
» perch (orange roughy)
» barramundi (larger fillets)
» gemfish
» large ling
» larger tuna (albacore, southern bluefin)

Do not eat frozen fish as this is ten times higher in histamines. Avoid prawns as they are treated with sulphite preservative (cooked prawns and shrimp may be preservative-free but you will need to check). While you have eczema, avoid smoked salmon and other smoked fish as they are highly acidifying and may contain chemicals and increased amines.

Storage and serving tips

» Fresh seafood needs to be kept on ice or refrigerated at all times.
» Fish can be lightly fried in oil, steamed or baked in the oven.
» Do not overcook fish as it toughens it. You will know the fish is beginning to be overcooked if white spots appear during cooking.

Serve fish with eczema-friendly salads, Steamed Fish Parcels with Mashed Potato (p. 172), Mashed Potato (p. 162) with beans and carrots; or on skewers.

6. Beetroot (beets)

Beetroot, also known as beets, is an important vegetable for eczema sufferers as it has strong alkalizing properties which boost liver detoxification of chemicals. Beetroot is abundant in antioxidants, folate and iron. It is a potent blood cleanser and research shows that beetroot consumption lowers blood pressure and reduces the risk of blood clots. Beetroots are a rich source of betaine, a derivative of choline, which helps to prevent fatty liver and boost detoxification of chemicals. Betaine also has the important role of converting homocysteine, a harmful substance, into methionine, which is essential for proper liver function.[1]

Storage and serving tips

Beetroots last for weeks if stored in the refrigerator in a sealed plastic bag with a paper towel to absorb excess moisture.

Grate fresh, peeled beetroot into salads or salad sandwiches and use beetroot in freshly made vegetable juices. Do not consume canned beetroot as it contains vinegar. Recipes include Healthy Skin Juice (p. 187) and Banana Beet Smoothie Bowl (p. 193).

Note: beetroot contains moderate amounts of salicylates so if you have *severe* salicylate intolerance you may need to avoid consuming beetroot until your tolerance level improves. Avoid beetroot leaves as they are a rich source of salicylates.

7. Oats

Eczema sufferers need to start their day with a nutritious breakfast and wholegrain or rolled oats provide more dietary fibre and protein than other grain cereals. They're a source of vitamin E, zinc, potassium, iron, manganese and silica, an essential mineral for strengthening connective tissue in the skin. Oats contain soluble fibre, so when they're made into porridge it appears gluey during cooking. The fibre is valuable for gastrointestinal health, helping to lower cholesterol, promote liver health, and cleanse pathogens and toxin-loaded bile from the bowel.

Storage and serving tips

» Oats contain gluten because of cross contamination, as oats are usually grown near wheat crops and processed alongside wheat. Wheat-free (gluten-free) oats are available but alternatively you can soak your oats overnight to make the gluten easier to digest and this also reduces the phytic acid content.

» Store oats in a sealed container in a cupboard.

» If you are allergic or sensitive to oats you don't have to eat them — choose alternative recipes in this book.

Oat recipes include Raw Omega Muesli (granola) (p. 193), New Anzac Cookies (p. 182), and Wholegrain Oat Porridge (p. 142). If you are gluten intolerant make Quinoa Porridge (p. 144) as an alternative.

8. Papaya (and pawpaw)

Papaya is a red fruit related to yellow pawpaw and it provides a range of carotenoids, which are potent antioxidants that can modulate gene activity to protect against inflammatory damage and tumour growth, according to clinical studies.[2]

The lycopene content in papaya helps to protect the skin from sun damage (note that there is no lycopene in pawpaw) and both fruits are rich sources of vitamin C. Papaya contains the digestive enzyme papain, which is used in some digestive supplements to aid protein digestion. Papain kills parasites in the gut and after antibiotic use or a bout of illness you can eat a serving of papaya daily to promote recolonization of beneficial bacteria in the gastrointestinal tract.

Papaya is usually eaten raw, with the skin and seeds removed. The seeds contain potent antimicrobial properties and they can be eaten to flush worms out of the bowel ('flush' being the operative word as they cause severe diarrhoea, so use with caution and do not give papaya seeds to children). Eating papaya flesh does not cause any of these symptoms, although the fruit does contain a moderate amount of amines so if you are highly sensitive to amines make sure you're also taking a vitamin C, B6 and calcium supplement.

Note: papaya and pawpaw are considered low in salicylates. Both contain moderate amounts of amines so if you are highly sensitive to amines avoid both papaya and pawpaw.

Storage and serving tips

» If papaya is not available, use pawpaw in the recipes. Pawpaw is a similar fruit with yellow flesh and is often rounder and less sweet (see the 'Specialty ingredients' image on p. 51).

» Always buy your fruits whole, not pre-cut, as cut fruit can develop bacteria when cut.

» Ripen papaya or pawpaw on the kitchen bench, then store in the refrigerator as they can perish quickly once ripe. Cover in plastic wrap once cut.

Recipes include Papaya Rice Paper Rolls (p. 208), Papaya Nice Cream (p. 216), Healthy Skin Smoothie (p. 185), and Wholegrain Oat Porridge (p. 142).

9. Saffron

Saffron is a highly prized spice thanks to its medicinal properties, pleasant flavour and bright orange colour which is commonly used to colour rice dishes. Saffron has many health benefits and it has been used for centuries as a natural antiseptic, digestive aid and antidepressant. For people with digestive issues, adding saffron to your dishes may reduce your symptoms. Saffron also has anti-inflammatory properties and can be an effective remedy for stomach disorders and coughs thanks to the compounds safranal and crocin.[3]

Storage and serving tips

» Store saffron in a sealed container in a dark cupboard, as light can damage the pigment and flavour.

» A pinch of saffron is all that is needed in cooking.

» A few strands can be added to rice dishes during cooking.

» Saffron can also be added to desserts such as Papaya Nice Cream (p. 216) and Banana Nice Cream (p. 216) or Saffron Tea (p. 128).

10. Pears

Pears are a member of the rose family and have a unique combination of insoluble and soluble fibre. This powerful combination of dietary fibre in pears helps to reduce the risk of inflammatory diseases, heart disease and type 2 diabetes, by binding to bile acids to aid the removal of toxic waste from the body. Pears are a good source of vitamin C and vitamin K, and the flavonols in pears include quercetin and kaempferol, which are potent anti-inflammatory antioxidants with antifungal and anticancer properties. Pears are one of the few low acid, low-salicylate fruits making them gentle on the digestive tract and easier to digest than other fruits.

Storage and serving tips

» Pears are generally bought unripe and perish quickly once ripe, because they are low in salicylates which act as a preservative. So leave them on the bench to ripen and refrigerate them when they are ready.

» To test if a pear is ripe, press at the very top of the pear around the stem and if the spot gives with pressure it is ripe (the rest of the pear may feel firm).

» If you want to speed up the ripening process, store the pears together in a large brown paper bag at room temperature. Once they are ripe, if you want to slow down the ripening process store them separately in open plastic bags in the refrigerator.

» Once peeled and cut, pears can quickly oxidize (go brown) so consume them immediately or stew them briefly in boiling water to retain the colour.

Recipes include Pink Pear Jam (p. 137), Pear and Vanilla Tea (p. 126) and Pear Crumble (p. 178).

11. Carob

Carob has been used for its many health benefits for over 4000 years. It was used to soothe and cleanse the throat and it can help alleviate diarrhoea in children.

Carob is naturally caffeine-free and sweeter tasting than cocoa so it requires little or no sugar to taste good. It improves digestion, contains anti-cancer compounds and it supplies calcium, magnesium, vitamin B2 and B6, dietary fibre and more.

According to the *Encyclopedia of Healing Foods*, carob contains tannins, however they are not the anti-nutrient kind. Unlike many tannins, the ones in carob are not water soluble so they do not bind to proteins and render them unavailable. And the tannins in carob also have several beneficial effects, including binding to toxins to inactivate them and inhibiting the growth of bacteria.

Carob also curbs hunger as it inhibits the hormone ghrelin, which makes you feel hungry. According to research, ghrelin levels in saliva are significantly elevated in patients with atopic eczema (compared with eczema-free people). This can make eczema sufferers feel hungry at bedtime or during the night, which promotes broken sleep and can make it difficult falling asleep at night. So having a cup of Carob Tea (p. 126) before bed can help to promote satiety and better quality sleep.

Storage and serving tips

» Pure carob can be bought in powder form, as nibs or syrup, from selected health food stores.

» Store it in an airtight container in a dark cupboard.

» When cooking a recipe that includes cocoa or cacao (both are high in amines and not permitted on the diet), you can substitute these ingredients with raw carob powder.

Use carob in recipes such as Carob Tea (p. 126), Carob Syrup (p. 134) and Protein Smoothie Bowl (p. 194).

12. Potatoes

While potatoes are often mistakenly touted as being 'void of nutrition' this humble vegetable has a high vitamin C content, which kept sailors in the 1700s from dying of scurvy. White potatoes are a rich source of antioxidants and vitamin B6, and a good source of potassium, magnesium, copper, manganese, vitamin B5 and dietary fibre for healthy bowels and clear skin. White potatoes also contain valuable antioxidants including alpha lipoic acid, which helps the body control blood sugar levels, and choline, an exceptional B-vitamin like nutrient, which helps to reduce inflammation and break down fats in the liver.

Storage and serving tips

» As potato skin contains salicylates, during the Eczema Detox and FID programs all potatoes should be peeled to reduce the salicylate content.

» Sweet potato contains medium amounts of salicylates so if you are not sensitive to salicylates then sweet potato can be added to your diet in the Eczema Detox Program.

» Store potatoes in a potato jar in a dark cupboard. When stored correctly, in cooler weather potatoes can last for a month or more; however, use them quickly as the skins can develop green patches which should not be consumed.

» If you are allergic or sensitive to potatoes, you can avoid this ingredient.

Peeled potatoes can be mashed, baked or lightly fried. Recipes include New Potato and Leek Soup (p. 163) and Steamed Fish Parcels with Mashed Potato (p. 172).

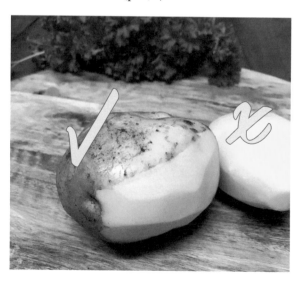

White versus cream potatoes — choose white

Chapter 6
Other useful ingredients

This chapter features some further useful ingredients for those with skin rashes and possible chemical intolerances, including eczema-friendly cooking oils, sweeteners and non-dairy milks. On p. 51 there's also a photo of some of the specialty ingredients used in the programs, so you know exactly what to look for when at the supermarket.

Raw cashews

Cashews are rich in skin-supporting minerals including manganese, magnesium and zinc. A quarter of a cup (about 40 g) of cashews supplies 98 per cent of the recommended daily intake (RDI) of copper. Copper is an important component of the enzyme superoxide dismutase, which plays a critical role in reducing inflammation and detoxifying chemicals via the liver. Cashews have a lower fat content than most nuts, with 80 per cent unsaturated fatty acids, most being the heart-healthy monounsaturated fats like the ones found in extra virgin olive oil.

Why choose raw? Roasted cashews develop amines and salicylates so buy the raw cashews as they are free of these chemicals.

What are activated cashews?

Nuts and seeds contain small amounts of phytates, which bind to minerals such as iron and zinc. This is not normally an issue if your body's gut bacteria adequately break down the phytic acid. However, if you have digestive problems or skin inflammation it's a good idea to 'activate' your nuts before use. Activating nuts is an ancient practice where nuts are soaked in mildly salty water and (traditionally) dried in the sun.

How to activate cashews

You will need:

- 1 or 2 cups of raw cashews (whatever amount required)
- sprinkle of quality sea salt
- enough water to cover

Place the ingredients into a container, remove any damaged or discoloured cashews and cover with a lid. Allow to soak for about 4 hours or overnight. Do not soak them for longer. Then strain and discard the water and rinse the cashews well. If you are using the nuts for making Cashew Nut Butter (p. 189) or Cashew Nut Milk (p. 184), then there is no need to dry out the nuts.

If you wish to dry the nuts, using an oven may result in the nuts developing amines (which is fine if you are not sensitive to amines but you won't know this until you have done the test on p. 84. However, you can dry the nuts with a paper towel then place them in a container covered with mesh or cloth (sealed to prevent visitors), and place on a sunny windowsill for 24 hours or until dry.

Caution is advised when consuming cashews. If you are sensitive to nuts, avoid cashews. If you are unsure if you react to cashews, test them in week 3 of the FID Program. It is important to test them — if you adversely react to cashews but continue to eat them you could prevent your eczema from clearing up. Testing them gives you clarity so you can safely eat them or avoid them if necessary (testing instructions are on p. 84).

Eczema-friendly cooking oils

» rice bran oil

» sunflower oil

» refined safflower oil

Rice bran oil is low in salicylates and, like olive oil, contains oleic acid and vitamin E — 1 tablespoon supplies about 40 per cent of the RDI for vitamin E. Rice bran oil contains some omega-3 and double the amount of omega-6 essential fatty acids, which should only be consumed in moderation. It also contains gamma-oryzanol, a powerful antioxidant and plant sterol that reduces the absorption of cholesterol. Rice bran oil also has one of the highest smoking points so it's one of the safest oils to use when frying or baking.

If you are allergic to rice or sensitive to rice bran oil (it is rare but possible), then avoid rice bran oil and use other eczema-friendly oils that are salicylate-free including refined sunflower oil and refined safflower oil *but check there is no antioxidant and no additives in these oils!*

Remember: it's still important to reduce your oil and fat intake and only use cooking oils in moderation. You do not need to consume cooking oil in this diet — rice bran oil is an optional ingredient.

Oils to avoid

Avoid consuming olive oil, coconut oil, almond oil and other nut oils as they are rich sources of itch-promoting salicylates. I am not saying these oils are bad in general — they are rich in salicylates which are off limits for now. Once your eczema completely clears up you might like to test your favourite oil to see if you can tolerate it without an adverse reaction.

Margarine and butter

Margarines must be strictly avoided, even the dairy-free ones, as they contain itch-prompting additives including flavourings, vitamin A and artificial antioxidants that worsen eczema. The research shows families who frequently use margarine are more likely to have a child who develops eczema by age two.[1,2,3]

Butter is a dairy product that often contains additives and oils to soften it, so it must be strictly avoided (for now). *Once your eczema completely clears up*, and if you are not allergic to dairy products, you might like to test pure ghee (clarified butter) or pure organic butter that contains no oils or additives.

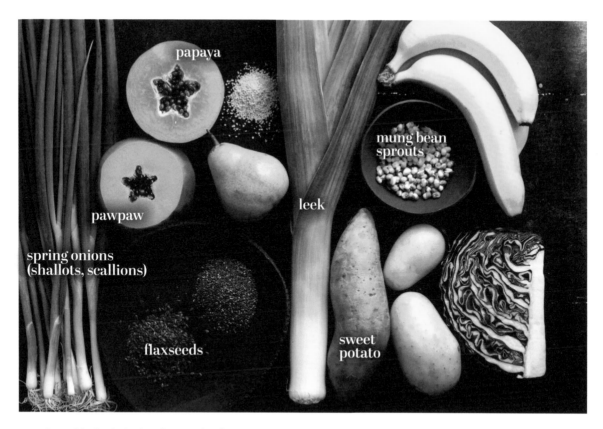

Some of the skin-loving ingredients used in the Eczema Detox and FID programs, including spring onions (also known as shallots or scallions), papaya, mung bean sprouts, flaxseeds and chia seeds.

Tips for a balanced diet

When following any of the programs in this book, follow these five tips to ensure you get a balanced diet:

1. Eat five servings of eczema-safe vegetables daily (p. 54)
2. Eat two pieces of eczema-safe fruit daily (p. 54)
3. Eat two to four servings of eczema-safe grains daily (p. 55)
4. Eat two servings of eczema-safe protein daily (p. 53).
5. If you are vegetarian or vegan you can add a plain, unflavoured non-dairy protein powder to your program (see p. 73 for pea protein details).
6. Drink six to ten glasses of filtered water daily (plus eczema-safe vegetable juices and soups).

Note: one serving equals ½ cup, so five servings of vegetables is approximately 2½ cups.

Eczema-friendly sweeteners

» rice malt syrup   » real maple syrup
   (brown rice syrup)   » barley malt

Ideally, your diet should have no added sweeteners, but for those of you who wish to use sweetener the best choice is rice malt syrup (which is known as brown rice syrup in the United States), as it is salicylate-free. Why this takes first preference is because it is the only alkalizing sweetener, as all other sweeteners convert to acid in the body.

In order of preference, the sweeteners eczema sufferers can use in recipes are:

»   rice malt syrup (alkalizing, low in chemicals)
»   real maple syrup (acid-producing, low in chemicals)
»   barley malt (acid-producing, low in chemicals, contains gluten).

Non-dairy milks

» cashew nut milk   » organic soy milk
» rice milk   » oat milk

As dairy products are pro-inflammatory in people with eczema and allergies, all animal milks (including cow, goat and sheep's milk) should be avoided while following the programs in this book. If you wish, you do not need to have a milk substitute — some people prefer to avoid all man-made milks and this is fine. However, if you would like dairy alternatives, favour the eczema-friendly milks listed here (remembering to continue to avoid the foods and drinks you are allergic to or suspect you are sensitive to).

For those of you who would like to consume milk in your porridge, smoothies and baked goods, here are the options to choose from:

» Cashew Nut Milk (p. 184)   » organic soy milk (with whole soybean, not poor quality 'soy isolate'; if you are gluten intolerant, choose malt-free soy milk)
» rice milk (check ingredients; sunflower oil is okay)   » oat milk (contains gluten).

Milks to avoid

Avoid almond milk, coconut milk and coconut water (for now) as they are rich sources of itch-promoting salicylates and amines. If you like these ingredients you can test them once your skin rash completely clears up. However, don't add these drinks back into your diet too soon as they could trigger your rash to return.

Choosing eczema-friendly alternatives

The following table lists some common foods and ingredients in the left column, along with eczema-friendly alternatives in the right column so you can swap foods to help your skin heal. Just be sure to avoid anything you're allergic to or have a sensitivity to.

Eczema-friendly alternatives

Swap this	For this! Choose from these ingredients
Oils: olive oil, extra virgin olive oil, coconut oil, almond oil and other nut oils, vegetable oils, peanut oil, canola oil etc.	Rice bran oil, brown rice oil, sunflower oil, refined safflower oil (no antioxidant additives, *not* extra virgin due to salicylate content)
Refined white sugar, raw sugar, brown sugar, molasses, artificial sweeteners, stevia, cocoa powder, honey, agave, corn syrup, coconut sugar, date sugar etc.	Rice malt syrup (brown rice syrup), real maple syrup, maple sugar, 100% carob syrup, carob powder, (another alternative: barley malt syrup) *Note: if you are sensitive to fructose you will need to avoid all syrups in this column
Dairy: cow/goat/sheep's milk, butter, milkshakes, cheeses, yoghurt, fermented dairy products, probiotics with dairy, dairy ice-creams, dairy ice lollies (popsicles), kefir etc.	Cashew Nut Milk (p. 184), rice milk, organic soy milk (whole soybean, not 'soy isolate'), oat milk, Cashew Nut Butter* (p. 189), Parsley Pesto* (p. 189), Banana Nice Cream* (p. 216), Papaya Nice Cream* (p. 216), calcium supplement (p. 70)
Pork, ham, bacon, beef, deli meats, sausages, mince with preservatives (not listed on packaging)	Lean lamb, free-range chicken, beef bones used in broth, lean minced lamb/veal/chicken (ask butcher for additive-free, freshly made mince)
Smoked salmon/fish, large fish such as flake and tuna (as they are rich in mercury), canned tuna in oil or olive oil	Baked or grilled fresh small white fish (see fish information on p. 78 and p. 92), fresh salmon may be consumed on the Eczema Detox Program (not FID Program)
Margarine, dairy-free margarine, softened butter (contains additives/oils), jams, spreads, avocado spread	Cashew Nut Butter* (p. 189), Sesame-free Hummus (p. 132), Parsley Pesto* (p. 189), Bean Dip (p. 132)

Swap this	For this! Choose from these ingredients
Raw egg white, whole-egg mayonnaise, dips containing egg	Egg Replacer (p. 211, also available in the supermarket baking section), Sesame-free Hummus (p. 132) instead of mayonnaise (when eczema improves: 1 free-range egg cooked, per week, if not allergic to egg)
Most fruits (they are rich in natural chemicals), fruit juices, avocado	Peeled pears (Eczema Detox Program also allows bananas, pawpaw and papaya)
Tomato, tomato-containing products, capsicum (bell pepper), mushrooms, pumpkin (winter squash), broccoli	Carrot, celery, potato, sweet potato, green beans, Brussels sprouts, cabbage (white and red)
Dark leafy greens, spinach, silverbeet (chard), rocket (arugula) etc.	Cos (romaine) lettuce*, iceberg lettuce (if you are on the FID Program favour iceberg lettuce)
Most herbs and all spices	Parsley (dried and fresh), chives (dried and fresh)
Onions, most sprouts	Leeks, spring onion (scallions, shallots), garlic, dried garlic powder, mung bean sprouts, lentil sprouts, sprouted spelt
Soy sauce/tamari, tomato sauce, barbecue sauce and other sauces, salad dressings of any kind	Cashew Nut Butter* (p. 189), Sesame-free Hummus (p. 132), Parsley Pesto* (p. 189), Bean Dip (p. 132), Maple Dressing (p. 135)
Dried fruits	Peeled pear, papaya*, pawpaw*, banana*
Most nuts	Unsalted raw cashews (if you are not allergic or sensitive to nuts)
Vinegar, pickled foods, gherkins (pickles)	Malt vinegar*, if you are not sensitive to salicylates (contains medium salicylates and may contain sulphites so don't add this ingredient into your diet until you have tested for salicylate and sulphite sensitivity in week 4 of the FID Program)

Swap this	For this! Choose from these ingredients
Wheat products, wheat flour, plain (all-purpose) flour, wheat bread, commercial wheat breakfast cereals, wheat pasta, jasmine rice, basmati rice	Spelt Flat Bread (p. 155), spelt flour, spelt sourdough, buckwheat, brown rice, low GI white rice, quinoa, rolled (porridge) oats, wheat-free oats, rice bran, brown rice flour/rice flour, barley, rye, potato flour, soy flour, rye flour, quinoa flour, plain gluten-free bread (highly refined cornflour may be okay if you are not sensitive to corn), gluten-free rice pasta, buckwheat pasta, Gluten-free Besan Pastry (p. 198)
Corn/maize (unrefined corn), corn cereals, corn chips	Plain brown rice crackers, plain salted rice crackers (no soy sauce, additives or seaweed etc.), plain puffed rice cereals, plain puffed quinoa cereals (caution: high GI), wholegrain rolled oats (no dried fruits or nuts; homebrand is usually best as it is less refined), refined/quick oats (caution: high GI so favour rolled oats)
Broad beans (fava beans)	Other beans, kidney beans, navy beans, lentils, cannellini beans, chickpeas (garbanzo beans), green beans
Soft drink (sodas), diet soft drink, flavoured or coloured mineral water, tap water	Filtered water, natural springwater (no colours or flavours), plain mineral water, Electrolyte Pear Juice (p. 128)
Coffee, teas, herbal teas, fruit juices	Carob Tea (p. 126), Pear and Vanilla Tea (p. 126), Healthy Skin Smoothie (p. 185), Celery Cleansing Juice (p. 125)
Biscuits (cookies), muffins, snack foods, cakes, pastries, chips (crisps), pancake mix, confectionery/lollies/candy, chocolate, cocoa/cacao	Pear Spelt Muffins (p. 151), Spelt Pancakes (p. 141), Mung Bean Sprout Pancakes (p. 168), plain rice crackers or rice cakes (no additives), Banana Bread* (p. 212), New Anzac Cookies (p. 182)

*Recipes/ingredients marked with an asterisk are for the Eczema Detox Program, not the FID Program (but they can be tested in the FID Program in weeks 3–4).

PART 3
programs and menus

Chapter 7
Skin Supplement Program

A range of nutrients work together to repair, renew and moisturize your skin. These are covered in detail in this chapter.

Here are the top 11 nutients for helping alleviate eczema and skin inflammation:

1. vitamin B6
2. biotin
3. magnesium
4. vitamin C
5. zinc
6. omega-3
7. taurine
8. molybdenum
9. calcium
10. vitamin D
11. protein

For other skin disorders and chemical intolerances, refer to the information in this chapter plus the skin disorder chart on pp. 31–5. If you are following a vegetarian or vegan diet, three important supplements include:

» vitamin B12
» iron (if a blood test reveals you are low in iron)
» pea protein powder (see p. 73).

Note: this chapter does not contain every nutrient remedy as it caters to skin disorders. If the nutrient you would like information on does not appear in this book, then head to www.eczemalife.com and use the search box to search for the particular nutrient.

1. Vitamin B6

Vitamin B6 is essential for healthy skin and a normal functioning immune system. It is a natural antihistamine with the ability to reduce histamine intolerance (along with vitamin C), making it helpful for people with allergies and histamine intolerance. Vitamin B6 helps the liver detoxify chemicals and it can reduce the toxic effects of salicylates, benzoic acids, food preservatives, monosodium glutamate (MSG), alcohol and heavy metals. Vitamin B6 is essential for normal fat metabolism and, as a result, a *deficiency* in vitamin B6 can raise cholesterol levels and cause fatty liver.[1]

Vitamin B6: dosages and food sources

Vitamin B6 (also known as)	Supplement dosages (milligrams per day)	Eczema-friendly food sources
Pyridoxine Pyridoxamine Pyridoxal Pyridoxine hydrochloride Pyridoxal-5-phosphate	**Infants (AI)** 0.1–0.3 mg from breastmilk or hypoallergenic (dairy-free) infant formula **Children + teens** 1–4 years: 0.5–3 mg 5–12 years: 1–6 mg 13–18 years: 1.3–6 mg **Adults** RDI: 1.3–2 mg Therapeutic: 6–10 mg	150 g (5 oz) grilled salmon: 1.2 mg* 1 medium potato: 0.7 mg 1 cup sweet potato: 0.6 mg^ 1 cup mashed potato: 0.5 mg 1 cup cooked lentils: 0.45 mg 150 g (5 oz) cooked beef: 0.44 mg 150 g (5 oz) cooked chicken/turkey: 0.4 mg 100 g (3½ oz) Brussels sprouts: 0.37 mg 1 medium banana: 0.35 mg* 80 g (3 oz) buckwheat: 0.32 mg 1 fillet (127 g) flatfish/flounder: 0.3 mg 60 g (2½ oz) rolled (porridge) oats: 0.19 mg 30 g (1 oz) raw cashews: 0.16 mg

AI: Adequate Intake as per Australian Government guidelines.
RDI: Recommended Daily Intake as per Australian Government guidelines, shown on the table as the lowest dose. The higher range covers the therapeutic range.
^Contains salicylates (not suitable during weeks 1–3 of the FID Program)
* Contains amines

Note: as B-group vitamins are acidic, avoid mega-doses above 15 mg. In order to prevent deficiencies of other B vitamins, take vitamin B6 in supplement form along with other B vitamins, not as a single supplement.

2. Biotin

Biotin is essential for skin health and normal hair growth. Since the 1950s it has been well established that biotin deficiency can cause eczema and dermatitis. While not all cases are caused by biotin deficiency, this B-group vitamin is an essential part of any treatment program for skin inflammation. Biotin from food sources is usually attached to protein and is poorly absorbed by the body.

Egg white injury (biotin deficiency)

It's important to avoid eating raw egg whites. 'Egg white injury' can occur when avidin, a protein in raw egg whites, latches onto biotin so your body cannot use it. Skin inflammation is one of the first signs of this happening. While eating raw eggs occasionally won't cause egg white injury, avoid consuming egg protein smoothies, pavlova, some dips, chocolate mousse and mayonnaise — these foods are bad for eczema.

Biotin: dosages and food sources

Biotin (also known as)	Supplement dosages (micrograms per day)	Eczema-friendly food sources
Vitamin B7 Vitamin H	**Infants (AI)** 5–6 mcg from breastmilk or hypoallergenic (dairy-free) infant formula **Children +teens** 1–4 years: 8–30 mcg 5–12 years: 20–60 mcg 13–18 years: 30–60 mcg **Adults** 30–90 mcg	1 cup cooked soybeans: 40 mcg 1 egg: 15 mcg (avoid raw egg) 150 g (5 oz) grilled salmon: 14 mcg* 60 g (2⅓ oz) oats: 12 mcg 1 cup sweet potato: 8.6 mcg^ 1 cup carrots: 6 mcg^ 1 medium banana: 3 mcg* (biotin is poorly absorbed from foods) (mcg is also referred to as μg)

AI: Adequate Intake as per Australian Government guidelines, shown on the table as the lowest dose (no set RDIs). The higher range is the therapeutic dose. ^Contains salicylates (not suitable during weeks 1–3 of the FID Program).
*Contains amines (not suitable for weeks 1–2 of the FID Program).

Note: take biotin with vitamin B6, magnesium and zinc to reduce skin inflammation, as they aid the conversion of omega-6 and omega-3 fats to healthy, anti-inflammatory substances.

3. Magnesium

Magnesium supplementation is important as it can decrease food chemical intolerances when combined with taurine, calcium carbonate and vitamin B6. The ability for your body to absorb magnesium naturally declines as you age and magnesium deficiency is common. It can be caused by diarrhoea, poor diet, low protein diets (less than 30 g/1 oz per day), fat malabsorption, frequent alcohol consumption, and frequent use of antibiotics or diuretics.

Note: if you are following the FID Program or any other program in this book, do not combine this supplement routine with herbal preparations or supplements containing fruit flavourings or vegetable extracts as they are rich in salicylates, which can prevent your low-chemical program from being effective. To make it easier for you to find suitable low-salicylate supplements there are product recommendations in 'Useful resources' on p. 220, and refer to the Skin Supplement Program table at the end of this chapter.

Nutrients for depression

In order for your body to produce the feel-good chemicals serotonin and dopamine, your body needs taurine and co-factors including vitamin B6, vitamin B12, folate, magnesium and zinc. Omega-3 is also important for healthy brain function (see omega-3 information on p. 64).

Magnesium: dosages and food sources

Magnesium (also known as)	Supplement dosages (milligrams per day)*	Eczema-friendly food sources
Magnesium carbonate (good, highly alkaline) Magnesium bisglycinate (good form, contains glycine) Magnesium orotate (most expensive, well absorbed) Magnesium citrate (less alkaline due to citric acid) Magnesium oxide (poorly absorbed)	**Infants (AI)** 30–75 mg from breastmilk or hypoallergenic/dairy-free infant formula **Children + teens** 1–4 years RDI: 80 mg (40–65 mg from supplement) 5–12 years RDI: 130–240 mg from food (80–130 mg from supplement) 14–18 years RDI: 410 mg (120–200 mg from supplement) **Adults** RDI: 310–400 mg (120–200 mg from supplement)	1 cup soybeans: 148 mg 1 cup black beans: 120 mg ¼ cup raw cashews: 117 mg 1 cup cooked spelt: 95 mg 1 cup navy beans: 96.5 mg 1 cup buckwheat: 85.7 mg 60 g (2½ oz) raw oats: 80 mg 1 cup cooked brown rice: 83 mg ⅓ cup barley: 81 mg 1 fillet (127 g) flathead/flounder: 74 mg 1 cup cooked dried beans: 75 mg 100 g (3½ oz) canned sardines: 60 mg^ 1 cup sweet potato: 54 mg^ fish (average serving): 26–50 mg ½ cup tofu: 47 mg ½ papaya: 26 mg^ 1 cup mashed potato: 38 mg 1 cup Brussels sprouts: 31 mg 1 cup boiled skinless potatoes: 31 mg chicken or red meat (average serving): 30 mg 1 cup mung bean sprouts: 22 mg ½ cup leeks: 7 mg ½ cup celery: 5 mg

*Plus consume magnesium from food sources
AI: Adequate Intake as per Australian Government guidelines.
RDI: Recommended Daily Intake from foods as per Australian Government guidelines shown on the table as the highest dose. The lower range is the recommended dose in supplements as you should also consume magnesium via a healthy diet.
^Contains salicylates (not suitable during weeks 1–3 of the FID Program).

Notes:
- Take magnesium more than 2 hours apart from medications.
- Take magnesium along with vitamin B6, taurine and calcium carbonate.

4. Vitamin C

Vitamin C (also known as ascorbic acid) is vital for the formation of collagen in the skin and it is necessary for wound healing. It is a natural antihistamine, as vitamin C destroys the imidazole ring of the histamine molecule. Vitamin C deficiency can result in histamine toxicity and as a consequence allergic reactions may increase in severity. If you have allergies and eczema it's essential to take extra vitamin C.

Vitamin C: dosages and food sources

Vitamin C (also known as)	Supplement dosages (milligrams per day)	Eczema-friendly food sources
Ascorbic acid Calcium ascorbate Magnesium ascorbate (avoid: it contains sulphites) Sodium ascorbate	**Infants (AI)** 25–30 mg from breastmilk or hypoallergenic (dairy-free) infant formula **Children + teens** 1–4 years: 35–70 mg 5–12 years: 40–140 mg 14–18 years: 40–210 mg **Adults** 60–210 mg	100 g (3½ oz) Brussels sprouts: 110 mg 150 g (5 oz) papaya or pawpaw: 90 mg* 100 g (3½ oz) cabbage: 45 mg 100 g (3½ oz) leek: 30 mg 100 g (3½ oz) sweet potato: 25 mg^ 100 g (3½ oz) swede/rutabaga/turnip: 25 mg 1 medium potato: 30 mg 100 g (3½ oz) green beans: 20 mg 1 banana: 15 mg* 1 cup mung bean sprouts: 14 mg 3 spring onions (scallions, shallots): 15 mg 10 g (⅓ oz) parsley: 10 mg

AI: Adequate Intake as per Australian Government guidelines.
RDI: Recommended Daily Intake as per Australian Government guidelines, shown on the table as the lowest dose. The higher range is the therapeutic dose. As vitamin C is acidic, do not take high doses (above 250 mg).
^Contains salicylates (not suitable during weeks 1–3 of the FID Program).
*Contains amines (not suitable for weeks 1–2 of the FID Program).

Note: as vitamin C is acidic, consume it with an alkaline mineral such as magnesium carbonate or calcium carbonate.

5. Zinc

Zinc is vital for skin repair and maintenance. It inhibits histamine release so it can help to reverse histamine intolerance, along with vitamin B6, copper and vitamin C.[2] During teenage years, rapid development requires zinc and these growth spurts can lead to zinc deficiency, and as the skin's oil gland activity is regulated by zinc, acne can result. Zinc deficiency can lead to skin lesions, dry and rough skin and delayed wound healing. Severe zinc deficiency can induce blister-like dermatitis, eczema and hair loss.

Zinc: dosages and food sources

Zinc (also known as)	Supplement dosages (milligrams per day)	Eczema-friendly food sources (cooked)
Zinc gluconate (best form, absorbed well) Zinc picolinate* Zinc oxide (poorly absorbed)	**Infants (AI)** 2–3 mg from breastmilk or hypoallergenic (dairy-free) infant formula **Children + teens** 1–4 years: 3–5 mg 5–12 years: 6–10 mg 14–18 years: 7–15 mg (girls); 13–20 mg (boys) **Adults** Women: 8–15 mg Men: 14–20 mg	6 oysters: 27 mg** 150 g (5 oz) lamb shank: 14.5 mg 150 g (5 oz) beef: 7.7 mg 150 g (5 oz) lamb: 6.4 mg 100 g (3½ oz) dried beans: 3 mg 1 cup cooked spelt: 2.4 mg 100 g (3½ oz) raw brown rice: 2.1 mg 60 g (2½ oz) wholegrain oats: 1.1 mg 100 g (3½ oz) raw white rice: 1.1 mg 1 fillet (127 g) flathead/flounder: 0.8 mg ½ fillet (180 g) cooked salmon: 0.8 mg** 1 cup mashed potato: 0.6 mg 1 cup sweet potato: 0.6 mg^

AI: Adequate Intake as per Australian Government guidelines.
RDI: Recommended Daily Intake as per Australian Government guidelines, shown on the table as the lowest dose. The higher range is the therapeutic range.
^Contains salicylates (not suitable during weeks 1–3 of the FID Program).
**Contains amines (not suitable for weeks 1–2 of the FID Program).
*Note: I no longer recommend zinc picolinate. It is highly absorbable and as a result it can lead to zinc toxicity symptoms including vomiting, nausea, metallic taste in mouth and copper deficiency.

Notes:
- Salt, calcium, iron and phosphorus can prevent zinc supplements from being absorbed, so have your zinc-containing supplement more than 2 hours apart from these substances.
- Take zinc with vitamin B6, biotin and magnesium to help reduce skin inflammation.

6. Omega-3

Omega-3 is an incredible essential fatty acid (EFA) which is vital for healthy and hydrated skin that is rash-free. Rich sources of omega-3 include flaxseeds/linseeds, salmon, fish oils and chia seeds. In healthy people, omega-3 is converted into active forms that the body can easily use, including eicosapentaenoic acid (EPA) and docosahexaenoic acid (DHA). EPA and DHA help to block inflammation in the body, so ensure you are consuming enough omega-3.

Flaxseed oil research

Scientists De Spirt and colleagues gave two groups of women either flaxseed oil or borage oil for twelve weeks, and a third group received a placebo, which was olive oil. After six weeks of consuming only half a teaspoon of either flaxseed oil or borage oil, skin water loss was decreased by about 10 per cent, and by week twelve the flaxseed oil group showed further protection from water loss and the skin was significantly more hydrated. While the olive oil (placebo) group had no significant change in skin health, at *twelve weeks of use* the flaxseed oil group had significantly less skin reddening (after irritation), roughness and scaling of the skin.[3]

Note: vegetarian sources of omega-3 are mostly *unconverted*, with the exception of some types of algae, so this is shown in the first table. The next table shows the foods which have the *converted* forms — DHA and EPA; these are mostly seafoods that have consumed omega-3 rich algae. Note that EPA and DHA can be consumed in lower doses as they are in a form the body can readily use. This does not mean fish oils are better than flaxseed oil — I have seen many eczema sufferers benefit from using flaxseed oil.

Tip: to help the omega-3 in flaxseed oil convert into EPA, consume it with vitamin B6, biotin, magnesium and zinc (refer to Skin Supplement Program table, p. 75).

Notes:
- Omega-3 fish oil supplements thin the blood so discontinue use several weeks before surgery or childbirth.
- If you are following the FID Program, do not consume fish oil, chia seeds or flaxseed meal during weeks 1–2 as these products are tested in weeks 3–4. Alternatively, you can have ½ teaspoon of flaxseed oil daily as people with chemical sensitivity usually tolerate this low dose.
- If you are not allergic to fish, you can eat it one to three times per week (not more than three times per week).

Omega-3: dosages and food sources

Omega 3 (also known as)	Supplement dosages (milligrams per day)*	Eczema-friendly food sources
Alpha linolenic acid (ALA), also known as: Linolenic acid Note: take vitamin B6, biotin, zinc and magnesium to help convert ALA to EPA,	**Infants (AI)** 500 mg from breastmilk or hypoallergenic (dairy-free) infant formula **Children + teens** 1–3 years: 500–800 mg 4–8 years: 800–1000 mg 9–13 years: 1000–1500 mg 14–18 years: 1200–1800 mg **Adults** 1300–2000 mg	28 g (1 oz) flaxseeds: 6388 mg^* 28 g (1 oz) chia seeds: 4915 mg^* 1 tablespoon flaxseed oil: 7200 mg^* 1 teaspoon flaxseed oil: 2400 mg^* 1 cup soybeans: 700 mg 113 g (4 oz) tofu: 360 mg 1 cup cabbage: 170 mg

Omega-3: dosages and food sources

EPA/DHA (also known as)	Supplement dosages (milligrams per day)	Eczema-friendly food sources (EPA/DHA: the converted forms)
Eicosapentaenoic acid (EPA) and docosahexaenoic acid (DHA) Algae oil (vegan) Fish oil	**Infants (AI)** 20–30 mg from breastmilk or hypoallergenic (dairy-free) infant formula **Children + teens** 1–4 years: 40–200 mg 5–12 years: 70–250 mg 14–18 years: 85–500 mg **Adults** 160–1000 mg	100 g (3½ oz) Atlantic salmon: 1090–1830 mg^ 100 g (3½ oz) herring: 1710–1810 mg^ 100 g (3½ oz) sardines: 980–1700 mg^ 100 g (3½ oz) rainbow trout: 840–980 mg^ 100 g (3½ oz) mackerel: 340–1570 mg^ 150 g (5 oz) flathead: 300–400 mg 150 g (5 oz) John Dory: 200–300 mg

AI: Adequate Intake as per Australian Government guidelines, shown in the table as the lowest dose (there is no set RDI). The higher dose indicates the therapeutic range. Note larger fish such as flake, tuna and perch are rich in mercury so they are not included in this diet (mercury can worsen eczema).
^Contains amines (not suitable during weeks 1–2 of the FID Program).
*Contains salicylates (not suitable for weeks 1–3 of the FID Program).

Getting the omega balance right

Omega-6 is absolutely essential in the diet but too much can worsen eczema as it is used to make arachidonic acid in the body (the stuff that makes inflammation). Omega-6 is often consumed in excess in modern Western diets, with uneven ratios of about 16:1. According to asthma and arthritis research, to suppress inflammation the ideal ratio is between 3:1 and 5:1 (i.e. up to five times more omega-6 than omega-3).[4] The researchers noted that a ratio of 10:1 had adverse effects.

You can balance your essential fatty acid intake by consuming more omega-3 (from flaxseed oil) and less omega-6 from nuts, seeds and cooking oils and by avoiding margarine. The following table shows an example of what a balanced omega-3/omega-6 diet might look like. Keep in mind that avoiding all omega-6 is not the goal, as your body needs some omega-6 to prevent deficiency.

If an adult with eczema were to have a balanced daily intake of omega-6 and omega-3 (with a ratio of approximately 3:1), their diet could include the following:

Omega-3	Omega-6
(~2.4 g of omega-3) 1 teaspoon flaxseed oil (2.4 g omega-3 and 0.5 g omega-6) **If fresh fish is eaten twice a week, that would offer additional benefits (85 g/3 oz of salmon contains 2 g of total omega-3 or about 1 g of EPA/ DHA)	(~7.2 g of omega-6) 2 teaspoons rice bran oil* used in cooking, dressings and dips (3 g omega-6), plus ¼ cup raw cashews (2 g omega-6), plus minor sources of omega-6 such as meat, grains and fish (85 g/3 oz of salmon contains 0.5 mg of omega-6)

*If you are allergic or sensitive to rice bran oil, you may use small amounts of sunflower oil or safflower oil — these are salicylate-free oils. Note 1 teaspoon sunflower oil or safflower oil contains 3 g of omega-6, so they have double the amount of omega-6 so consume no more than 1 teaspoon per day or double the amount of omega-3 consumed from flaxseed oil. Note other oils are rich in salicylates and they are not a part of the program.
**As some people are allergic to fish, it was not included in the ratio calculations.

7. Taurine

Taurine is an incredible sulphur-containing amino acid which is required for liver detoxification of chemicals. Taurine is anti-inflammatory and helps to prevent tissue damage when inflammation occurs. People suffering from topical steroid withdrawal (TSW) often have excessively elevated nitric oxide levels in the blood and this can make them feel hot and itchy. Taurine helps to lower excess nitric oxide in the body, so taking taurine during TSW recovery can be beneficial.[5]

Taurine also assists with brain function. It is an important inhibitory neurotransmitter in the brain and it exerts an anti-anxiety and anti-stress effect.[6,7] Research shows that taurine levels can be significantly low in depressed patients.[8]

Taurine: dosages and food sources

Taurine (also known as)	Supplement dosages (milligrams per day)	Eczema-friendly food sources
Taurine (natural)	**Infants (AI)** 3–8 mg per 100 mls of breastmilk or hypoallergenic (dairy-free) infant formula **Children + teens** 1–4 years: 50–100 mg 5–12 years: 100–140 mg 14–18 years: 140–500 mg (plus food sources) **Adults** 200–500 mg per day Up to 2 g per day in divided doses	85 g (3 oz) cold-water fish: 120–400 mg 85 g (3 oz) chicken: 185 mg 85 g (3 oz) cooked red meat: 30mg

AI: Adequate Intake as per Australian Government guidelines.
No set RDIs available but research data shows doses up to 3 g (for adults) is safe.

Notes:
- Taurine supplementation helps to prevent fatty liver disease, which occurs in one-third of people with eczema.[9,10]
- Taurine deficiency can be tested via a whole blood test (not blood plasma, urine or stool tests as they are not as accurate).

8. Molybdenum

Eczema sufferers are commonly sensitive to sulphite-rich products including wine, grape juice and vinegar, and it could be due to molybdenum deficiency. Sulphite sensitivity signs also include hives, wheezing, asthma, discolouration of the skin, eczema, dermatitis, swelling, diarrhoea and anaphylaxis.[11] Deficiency signs of molybdenum include acne, allergies, asthma, rapid heart rate, sulphite intolerance, multiple chemical intolerances and sensitivity to mould and yeast.

How does sulphite sensitivity occur? Molybdenum plays an essential role in activating an enzyme called sulphite oxidase (SO), which plays a key role in breaking down sulphites in the liver.[12] Molybdenum helps the liver process sulphites, carbon and nitrogen and safely metabolizes drugs and toxins.[13] For example, if you have a *Candida albicans* infestation in your gut (from eating high-sugar foods), a toxin called acetaldehyde is produced during candida die-off. This toxin can cause fatigue, foggy brain function, joint pains and skin inflammation. However, taking molybdenum can reduce the adverse symptoms as it helps the liver to deactivate acetaldehyde.

Molybdenum: dosages and food sources

Molybdenum (also known as)	Supplement dosages (micrograms per day)	Eczema-friendly food sources
Molybdenum trioxide Molybdenum amino acid chelate	**Infants (AI)** 2–3 mcg from breastmilk or hypoallergenic (dairy-free) infant formula **Children + teens** 1–4 years: 17–22 mcg 5–12 years: 22–45 mcg 14–18 years: 34–67 mcg (girls); 43–67 mcg (boys) **Adults** 45–67 µg (up to 150 mcg) (mcg is also referred to as µg)	½ cup lentils: 74 mcg ½ cup dried peas: 73 mcg (avoid fresh peas) ½ cup lima beans: 70 mcg ½ cup soybeans: 64 mcg ½ cup black beans: 64 mcg ½ cup chickpeas (garbanzo beans): 61 mcg ¼ cup oats: 28 mcg 2 cups cos (romaine) lettuce: 5.6 mcg^ ⅓ cup barley: 26 mcg ½ cup chopped carrots: 3 mcg^ ½ cup chopped celery: 2.5 mcg

AI: Adequate Intake as per Australian Government guidelines (the RDI is the lower dose). The higher range is the therapeutic range.
^Contains salicylates (not suitable during weeks 1–3 of the FID Program).

Notes:
- Molybdenum is an essential mineral (i.e. your body does not make it) so you need to consume it in your diet. Molybdenum-rich foods are legumes, beans and lentils, so if you avoid these foods a deficiency can develop.[14]
- People with gastrointestinal disorders, such as Crohn's disease or gluten intolerance, can end up with molybdenum deficiency.[15]
- Take molybdenum along with taurine, vitamin B6, vitamin B5 and zinc to help your liver detoxify chemicals.

9. Calcium

Calcium is the most abundant mineral in the body and high levels are found in healthy, rash-free skin. Calcium deficiency signs include eczema, anxiety, hyperactivity, depression, heart palpitations and food sensitivities. Calcium boosts the acidity of the skin's acid mantle, which can increase the skin's ability to protect itself against dust mites and infections. Calcium also helps to maintain the right amount of moisturizing lipids in the epidermis layer of the skin by triggering lipid production.

Calcium carbonate is a salicylate sensitivity remedy as it is highly alkalizing and salicylate-free. It helps to quickly alkalize the blood and urine. Research shows the body eliminates excess salicylates *when the urine pH reaches 7.5* — and supplementing with calcium carbonate helps you reach this pH, which is how it temporarily reduces salicylate intolerance.

Calcium: dosages and food sources

Calcium (also known as)	Supplement dosages (milligrams per day)**	Eczema-friendly food sources
Calcium carbonate Calcium citrate* Calcium phosphate	**Infants (AI)** 210–270 mg from breastmilk or hypoallergenic (dairy-free) infant formula **Children + teens** 1–4 years: 200–500 mg 5–12 years: 400–1000 mg 14–18 years: 600–1000 mg **Adults** 600–800 mg	100 g (3½ oz) tofu: 350 mg 1 cup calcium-fortified soy milk or rice milk: 300 mg 100 g (3½ oz) sardines: 300 mg^ 100 g (3½ oz) salmon: 200–300 mg^ ½ cup green soybeans: 130 mg 1 bowl oatmeal/porridge: 99–110 mg ½ cup white beans: 96 mg 160 g (5 ⅓ oz) fish fillet: 85 mg 1 cup sweet potato: 76 mg^ 80 g (3 oz) rainbow trout: 73 mg^ 100 g (3½ oz) flathead/flounder: 23–55 mg 1 cup green beans: 55 mg 100 g (3½ oz) cabbage: 40 mg ½ cup celery: 20 mg 1 cup cooked spelt: 19 mg ½ cup leeks: 15 mg

AI: Adequate Intake as per Australian Government guidelines. The RDI is the higher dose, the lower dose is the amount to be taken in supplement form (obtain the remaining RDI via foods).

*Calcium citrate is not part of the program as it is mostly citric acid so it does not have the highly alkalizing effect of calcium carbonate.

**You should obtain the RDI of calcium from both supplements and non-dairy food sources.

^Contains salicylates so this ingredient is not suitable during weeks 1–3 of the FID Program.

Notes:
- Take calcium more than 2 hours apart from your medications, iron and zinc supplements.
- High calcium intake helps to block the absorption of lead and other harmful heavy metals.
- If you have an adverse reaction to salicylate-rich foods (for example after eating out), take a serving of Skin Friend PM to temporarily improve symptoms.
- Calcium deficiency can cause insomnia and poor sleep – so take calcium along with glycine and magnesium to promote a more restful night's sleep.

10. Vitamin D

Vitamin D is manufactured in the skin after exposure to direct sunlight, and is also obtained through your diet. Colleagues from the children's hospital in Boston have found that children with moderate to severe atopic eczema had significantly lower levels of vitamin D compared with children with milder symptoms. Deficiency is linked to a range of health problems including rickets, poor bone health, severe fatigue, psoriasis and muscle weakness. Deficiency signs of vitamin D include eczema or dermatitis, fatigue, joint pain or stiffness, psoriasis and muscle weakness.

Vitamin D: dosages and food sources

Vitamin D (also known as)	Supplement dosages (micrograms per day)	Eczema-friendly food sources
Cholecalciferol (vitamin D3) Note: Many vitamin D supplements are soy-based (see 'Useful resources' for suggestions)	**Infants (AI)** 5 mcg (200 IU) from breastmilk or hypoallergenic (dairy-free) infant formula **Children** 1–4 years: 5 mcg (200 IU) 5–12 years: 5–10 mcg (200–400 IU) **Adults** 5–20 mcg (400–800 IU) (IU = international units) (mcg is also referred to as µg)	100 g (3½ oz) grilled herring: 25 mcg^ 100 g (3½ oz) canned red salmon: 23.1 mcg^ 100 g (3½ oz) canned pink salmon: 17 mcg^ 150 g (5 oz) grilled trout: 16.5 mcg^ 150 g (5 oz) grilled salmon: 14.4 mcg^ 100 g (3½ oz) cooked kippers: 9.4 mcg 100 g (3½ oz) cooked mackerel: 5.4 mcg^ 100 g (3½ oz) flathead: 1 mcg

AI: Adequate Intake as per Australian Government guidelines.
RDI: Recommended Daily Intake as per Australian Government guidelines, shown on the table as the lowest dose. The higher range is the therapeutic dose.
^This ingredient contains amines so it is not permitted on the FID Program during weeks 1–2. Fresh white fish, such as flathead, is allowed on both programs if you are not allergic to seafood.

Notes:
  – Vitamin D can cause insomnia if taken late in the afternoon or before bed so consume it earlier in the day.
  – Frequent use of cortisone cream can deplete vitamin D levels in the skin.
  – As vitamin D is manufactured in the skin after sunlight exposure, frequent and small exposure to sunlight combined with a healthy diet and supplementation can help restore vitamin D levels.

11. Protein

If you are vegan, vegetarian, over age 60 or want to supplement your weight-training program with more protein, a suitable protein powder is pure pea protein *that has no flavourings or other ingredients.* As pea protein is low in cysteine and methionine and high in lysine (making it an incomplete protein), you can buy pea protein mixed with brown rice protein, as rice protein is high in cysteine and methionine and low in lysine, making it a superior complete protein.

Protein: dosages and food sources

Protein (also known as)	Supplement dosages (grams per day)	Eczema-friendly food sources (protein amount in grams)
(various amino acids)	**Infants (AI)** 10 g per day from breastmilk or hypoallergenic (dairy-free) infant formula **Children + teens (RDI)** 1–3 years: 14 g 4–8 years: 40 g 9–13 years: 35 g (girls); 65 g (boys) 14–18 years: 45 g (girls); 65 g (boys) **Adults (RDI)** Men: 64–81* g Women: 46–57* g (*the higher amount is for people over 70)	150 g (5 oz) chicken: 42 g 150 g (5 oz) beef or lamb: 40 g 150 g (5 oz) fish: 36 g 100 g (3½ oz) canned tuna or salmon: 24 g 1 egg: 6 g Vegan and vegetarian sources 1 cup soybeans: 28.6 g 25 g (0.8 oz) pea protein powder: 20 g 113 g (4 oz) tofu: 18 g 1 cup cooked lentils: 18 g 1 cup beans (kidney/black/lima): 15 g 1 cup chickpeas/garbanzo: 14.5 g ¼ cup oats: 6.6 g 100 g (3½ oz) pasta, cooked: 5 g 28 g (1 oz) raw cashews: 5 g

Notes:
- All protein powders are rich in glutamic acid so people with MSG sensitivity or glutamate sensitivity can adversely react to protein powders. If you react to any products, discontinue use and consume other food sources of protein.
- Protein is essential for healthy skin so check you are eating enough – not too much or too little.

FAQs

'Do I need to take all of these nutrients in separate formulas?'

Not if you don't want to. Molybdenum, vitamin C, taurine, biotin, magnesium, zinc, vitamin B6 and other B vitamins can be found in Skin Friend AM. Skin Friend PM contains calcium, magnesium and glycine.

'I'm taking medications and my doctor said I can't take supplements. Will this affect my results?'

It is easier to clear up eczema when you supplement your diet as it speeds up the healing process. If you are taking medications and your doctor has advised you to avoid taking supplements, then you can use the food charts in this chapter to ensure you are consuming enough of the right nutrients. Begin with the FID Program for four weeks then progress to the Eczema Detox Program.

'What about probiotics; do I need them?'

Probiotics can be useful after taking a course of antibiotics (as antibiotics kill the good bacteria as well as the bad) and they can help with some bowel issues. Note that probiotics are rich in amines and 35 per cent of eczema sufferers adversely react to amines, so there is a risk they can worsen eczema. If you wish to take probiotics (*L. rhamnosus* strain) they can be tested in week 3 of the FID Program (see p. 82 for details).

Note: if you want to know more about probiotics, hemp seed products, olive leaf extract, turmeric and other popular supplements go to www.eczemalife.com and search 'Eczema Supplement Review'. If you would like to read information about iron supplementation or MTHFR mutations (a genetic defect related to vitamin B12 and folate metabolism), go to www.eczemalife.com. If you are pregnant or breastfeeding, you can find specific supplement and diet information via the website.

12-week program

While some people experience quick results, it can take time to heal your body from the inside out, especially if you have frequently used topical steroids or immunosuppressants. This supplement program does not contain drugs or ingredients that only suppress inflammation (as the inflammation comes back if the treatment relies on suppression). So follow this nourishing supplement program for at least 12 weeks for best results. It is a safe program that can be followed long-term if needed.

More information

If you are after additional supplement information such as brands and stockists, see 'Useful resources' on p. 220.

Skin Supplement Program

When beginning this program for the first time, introduce one new product every three days. This supplement routine is a guide for healthy adults, teens and children (over age 1).

Morning (with breakfast, a snack or lunch)	Afternoon or night
1. Vitamin B6, biotin, vitamin C, taurine, zinc, molybdenum, magnesium, vitamin B12 etc. (Skin Friend AM), taken with food. Refer to package for dosages.	2. Calcium, magnesium and glycine (Skin Friend PM), taken with food. Refer to package for dosages.
3. Organic flaxseed oil (omega-3): taken with food at any time of the day. Begin with the lowest dose: · Children: ¼ to ½ teaspoon daily · Teens/adults: ½ to 1 teaspoon · Adults: ½ to 2 teaspoons If you are highly sensitive to amines or salicylates, keep the dosage at the lowest dose. Taking ½ teaspoon is usually well tolerated by sensitive individuals. Teens and adults can use capsules if preferred. If you adversely react to flaxseed oil, test other forms of omega-3.	Optional: fish (omega-3), if you are not allergic or sensitive to seafood, eat fresh fish (not frozen), 2–3 times a week (refer to fish information on p. 65).
Optional: vitamin D if you have been diagnosed with a deficiency (caution: vitamin D usually contains additives, check 'Useful resources', p. 220). Test this product separately to see if your skin is okay while using it.	Optional: pea/rice protein (no flavourings or additives) for vegetarians, vegans, the elderly and weight trainers. See the Protein Smoothie Bowl recipe (p. 194). Have a protein smoothie once or twice at any time of the day, especially after exercise.

This program does not take into consideration your personal health history and it may be unsuitable for pregnant women and people taking medical drugs.

Chapter 8
Food Intolerance Diagnosis (FID) Program

I found the elimination diet extremely helpful. Even though prior to this, I followed a very fresh, unprocessed plant-based diet with lots of vegetables and salads, my health and energy levels were not the best as I always felt sick and tired. Before seeing Karen, I had increased my intake of vegetables to five to seven serves a day and two pieces of fruit a day. I also avoided sugar, alcohol, caffeine, juices, soft drinks (sodas), dairy, gluten and packaged foods. But the 'healthier' I ate, the more bloated, itchy and tired I became. Stopping the foods I always ate during the elimination made me feel so much better. I started to feel better in a few days as my bloating, itchiness and acid reflux settled. If I'd never done the diet I would never have known. I recommend this elimination diet to anyone who feels stuck and frustrated. Two weeks on the elimination diet is easy.

JANA, AUSTRALIA

This chapter will give you all the information you need to follow the Food Intolerance Diagnosis (FID) Program. Let's start with a patient case study.

Case study: Jenny

Jenny is 28 years old and was diagnosed with eczema when she was only two months old and it never went away. As a child she had eczema on her elbows, wrists, behind her knees and on her neck. Then at age twenty she was diagnosed with a thyroid problem and after treatment her eczema worsened. Her eczema was now head to toe, very itchy and she couldn't sleep. At age 27, she began the Eczema Detox and noticed her skin became less itchy.

Then Jenny came to see me. Her skin would be good for a day and then it would flare up for no apparent reason. She realized her skin was worse when she was stressed. In a follow-up consultation I suggested she might have severe salicylate intolerance. So she took the remaining salicylate-containing foods out of her diet (a protocol on the FID

Program), including sweet potato, carrot, papaya and beetroot (beets), and her eczema cleared up after a week.

Jenny said:

> After 28 years of having eczema my skin is soft and smooth, I sleep through the night (as opposed to not sleeping at all), my relationships are better and I'm more confident. People say I look so much younger, healthier and happier. Hang in there, friends, I've been following Karen's diet for over a year now, and sometimes it's really, really hard. But after eight months on the diet my skin cleared up when I avoided salicylates. Then I reintroduced medium-salicylate foods, including beetroot, and my skin didn't react so I am becoming less sensitive to salicylates. I find now I occasionally get itchy skin if I go out with friends and eat regular food, but it doesn't break the skin. Previously it would welt as soon as I got itchy but not anymore. Now I have had a couple of big occasions where I've gone off the diet completely for the day … Tiny reaction on my hand the next day. But nothing else. Then I take an extra dose of Karen's supplements to help my skin recover faster.

Jenny's case is an example of how extra investigation can lead to the discovery of severe chemical sensitivity. As she had a lifetime of eczema to recover from, it took eight months but she was able to expand her diet to include beetroot (beets), snow peas (mangetout), asparagus, sweet potato, carrots and pumpkin (winter squash) — all are medium-salicylate foods — plus some spices which are high in salicylates. She still reacts to some high-salicylate foods including lemons and blueberries, and bananas cause raised, red welts on her skin so she avoids them. She is lactose intolerant so she continues to avoid dairy. She can safely eat cooked fish including salmon and tuna, which are good sources of omega-3. Jenny successfully completed the FID Program (Stage 1 and 2) and now follows the Eczema Detox Program and continues to expand her diet.

About the FID Program

The foods and drinks on the following list are low in salicylates and amines and free of natural MSG (glutamates). Note that a small number of these foods contain tannins, nitrates and goitrogens, so if you are sensitive to these chemicals avoid those foods during this test period. Remember, this is a *diagnostic program* designed to be restrictive for the first fourteen days to help you work out your trigger foods. I know it may seem daunting at first but it will help you to work out what your specific trigger foods are, so follow it strictly for the designated period of time.

FID Program food shopping list

The FID Program food shopping list in the following table outlines the foods you can eat when following the FID Program.

FID Program food shopping list (Stage 1: the elimination phase)[1,2,3,4]

Fruit
- [ ] peeled pears (T), pear (canned in sugar syrup, *not corn syrup or juice*)

Gluten-free
- [ ] arrowroot
- [ ] buckwheat
- [ ] gluten-free oats
- [ ] besan/chickpea/gram flour
- [ ] Doongara low GI rice
- [ ] white rice (*avoid jasmine and basmati rice*)
- [ ] plain puffed rice
- [ ] plain rice flakes
- [ ] white quinoa, quinoa flakes
- [ ] rice noodles (plain)

Gluten grains
- [ ] barley (G)
- [ ] rolled/wholegrain oats (G)
- [ ] rye (G)
- [ ] sourdough spelt bread (G; check it's wheat-free and no additives or yeast)
- [ ] spelt flour (G)

Vegetables
- [ ] bamboo shoots
- [ ] Beans, most (*not broad beans*)
- [ ] Brussels sprouts (O)
- [ ] white cabbage (O)
- [ ] red cabbage (O, T)
- [ ] celery (N)
- [ ] dried split peas (*not fresh peas*)
- [ ] green beans
- [ ] iceberg lettuce
- [ ] leeks
- [ ] mung bean sprouts
- [ ] white potato (e.g. Coliban, Kennebec, Sebago (*avoid: New, Baby, Dutch cream, Kipfler, Pontiac, Golden, Nicola, Desiree, coloured varieties*)
- [ ] shallots (spring onions, scallions)

Herbs/spices
- [ ] chives, fresh/dried
- [ ] garlic, fresh
- [ ] garlic powder
- [ ] parsley, fresh/dried
- [ ] saffron

Vegan protein
- [ ] beans (*not broad beans*), black beans (T), chickpeas/garbanzo beans, legumes, lentils (red/brown etc.)
- [ ] poppy seeds
- [ ] organic tofu (plain)

Animal protein
Fresh/not frozen, no preservatives
- [ ] beef
- [ ] chicken (skinless)
- [ ] fish (white only: flathead, hake, silver dory etc.)
- [ ] lamb
- [ ] rabbit
- [ ] veal

Beverages
plain, no seaweed, colours or flavours
- [ ] rice milk
- [ ] mineral water
- [ ] spring water
- [ ] organic soy milk

Flavourings
- [ ] carob powder (T)
- [ ] maple syrup (pure/real)
- [ ] pure carob syrup (T)
- [ ] rice malt syrup (brown rice syrup)
- [ ] sea salt (*no anti-caking agent*), Himalayan salt
- [ ] vanilla (real; T)

Oils
- [ ] rice bran oil/brown rice oil, (*if allergic to rice use safflower oil or sunflower oil, no antioxidant*)

Other
- [ ] carob nibs (e.g. Kibble Nibbles; T)

Note: You do not need to eat everything on this list. Avoid your allergy foods. Note that rye, millet, sago, swede (rutabaga) and barley malt are low in salicylates and fine to use but they are not in the recipes.
The following abbreviations indicate the presence of a particular chemical in a food:
(G) = gluten, (N) = nitrates, (O) = goitrogens, (T) = tannins

Eczema-friendly party treats

Here is a range of low-salicylate options for special occasions. Please note that sugar, fructose and alcohol (which is mostly sugar) are not good for eczema, so these treats are not recommended for daily consumption.

Eczema-friendly party treats

Party treats	Beverages	Alcohol
caramels (homemade)	decaf coffee (T) (no dairy)	(Note: all unflavoured and no preservatives)
potato crisps (plain salted, no flavours)	lemonade (plain clear, preservative-free)	gin
toffee (plain)		vodka
marshmallows, white (no colour)	**Desserts**	whiskey
New Anzac Cookies (p. 182)	Lemonade iceblocks/ice lollies/ popsicles (clear, no colour)	(mixed with soda water, plain mineral water or plain clear lemonade)

The 'itchy food' detective's diary

It is useful to keep a diet diary during this four-week test period. If you have a child with eczema, encourage them to become a 'food detective' by keeping a diet diary and rating their eczema at the end of each day.

» Help your child to understand why they are following this temporary diet program: to take away their 'itchies' and eczema.

» Encourage them to engage in their healing process by being a 'food detective' so they are less likely to sneak trigger foods when they are at school or a friend's house.

Unlike the Eczema Detox Program, which is more relaxed, the FID Program needs to be followed strictly or the results may be invalid. This program is not an 80/20 type of diet — you cannot accurately diagnose chemical sensitivities if you only follow it 80 per cent of the time. Once you have finished the four-week diagnosis period, you can have short breaks on the Eczema Detox Program, such as eating out and attending a social event. In the meantime, on pp. 80–4 I will give you instructions on how to follow the four-week FID Program from week to week.

Tips

Here are some tips to help you navigate your way through the FID Program.

Meats and seafood

For the first two weeks, meats and fish need to be freshly cooked, not leftovers, as leftovers develop amines. All meats should be fresh and not processed (i.e. not deli meat), and preferably organic. Frozen fish is high in amines so cannot be used during the two-week elimination period.

Season meats or white fish with quality sea salt, dried or fresh parsley, dried or fresh chives, fresh garlic and/or garlic powder. Avoid store-bought garlic paste or herb pastes as they may contain vinegar and other problematic ingredients that will affect your results.

Stocks and broth

Avoid all store-bought stock and bouillon, even freshly prepared stock, as they contain natural glutamates and amines that can affect your results. Use the Alkaline Vegetable Broth recipe on p. 167. If you pass the amine test in week three, there is a Therapeutic Broth recipe in this book on p. 205 which is suitable for flavouring soups and casseroles from week 4.

FID Program instructions (Stage 2: the testing phase)

The following instructions will guide you through each step of the four-week FID Program, helping you to uncover trigger foods and sensitivities.

FAQ

'How long does it take to see an adverse reaction?'

Allergic or sensitivity reactions *to a particular food* can take one to three days to develop, and *chemical intolerance* reactions can take up to ten days for obvious signs (but usually you will know within one to seven days). Adverse reactions can also be immediate. If you experience a worsening of symptoms, stop the test and wait until your flare-up subsides before beginning the next test. Test foods in the morning rather than at night so you can monitor reactions during daylight hours.

If you have asthma or anaphylaxis, medical supervision is advised and/or have your medications handy as you are allowed to use your asthma medications or EpiPen during the program. Do not test any foods you have an anaphylactic reaction to.

Common mistakes to avoid

- Don't abruptly stop using topical steroids or immunosuppressants during this four-week period as you may suffer withdrawal symptoms, which will confuse your results.
- Don't skip caffeine/sugar withdrawal week (pp. 21–2) as you need to do this separately.
- Ensure you are not eating leftover meats/fish as they develop amines from being refrigerated overnight after cooking — this is a common mistake that can affect your amine test results. Frozen fish is rich in amines and should be avoided.
- Don't accidentally eat the Eczema Detox Program recipes as they contain extra ingredients. Ensure the recipes you cook are labelled 'FID'.
- Don't do this test during periods of intense stress — ensure you are relatively calm and taking good care of yourself.
- Don't go hungry or leave cooking to the last minute. Take the time to prepare a range of recipes from this book as this will make the diet more enjoyable. There is plenty of food to eat if you cook in advance.
- If your skin clears up very quickly, don't be tempted to skip the testing phase. Take the time to identify the specific chemical/s that caused your eczema. For example, during testing you might react to salicylates and MSG but not amines, so you can expand your diet to include amine foods.
- Don't expect your skin to clear up within the two-week period. It can clear up within one to twelve weeks, but occasionally more investigation is required. Try to stay calm and be patient. Get plenty of rest and have ice packs handy during the testing phase to calm itchy skin.
- If you adversely react to FODMAPs, beans or fructose, don't eat them during this diet.
- Don't buy oils or products with additives such as antioxidant (refer to 'Additives to avoid' list on p. 102.
- Don't use antihistamine medications, as they will make food intolerance diagnosis unclear. If you are using antihistamine medications stop using them for a month. Once you know your trigger foods you won't need them again.
- You need to look for any kind of adverse symptoms, not just a worsening of eczema, such as a worsening of sinus problems, hay fever, headaches, hyperactivity etc. (refer to the chemical intolerance symptoms on p. 9).

Note: you are looking for patterns to see if you are reacting to a range of amine foods. It you suspect only one food it could indicate an allergy not amine intolerance.

Days 1 to 14: low-chemical diet

For two weeks, eat the foods on the FID Program food shopping list (p. 78), all of which are low amine and low salicylate. This food list must be followed strictly or the test will be invalid and you may need to begin again. Note how your skin looks and feels during these two weeks.

If you like, keep a diet diary to record your reactions to the new diet. Access a printable diet diary at www.eczemalife.com.

Days 15 to 21: test amines

Now comes the fun part. This week, test a range of amine-rich foods and note your reaction to each. You can change the order of foods to be tested (for example, if you want to test leftover meats, test leftovers first). You can combine several amine-rich foods within the week, as well as having a couple of 'very high amines' test days using dairy-free cocoa powder mixed into warm rice milk (do not test regular chocolate as it contains other ingredients).

Not everyone is sensitive to amines, which makes this a good test to complete first. If you already know you are sensitive to amines, skip this and move straight to the salicylate test.

How to test for amine intolerance:

Day 15: Eat 2–3 bananas (medium amounts of amines). Avoid small ladyfinger/sugar bananas as they contain salicylates (you will test salicylates next week). Try Banana Nice Cream (p. 216) with rice milk or eat fresh bananas. If you already know you are sensitive to bananas, skip to Day 16. If you have no adverse reactions continue to use banana for the duration of the test week.

Day 16: Eat 1 cup of fresh pawpaw and continue eating banana. If you have no reactions to eating pawpaw, continue eating it. Cook meat and save some for tomorrow's test.

Day 17: If you eat meat, introduce leftover meats (i.e. chicken or lamb) with lunch.

If you are vegetarian or vegan skip to Day 18 and repeat this day twice.

Days 18-19: Drink homemade hot chocolate (high amines). Buy pure 100 per cent cocoa powder — avoid cacao as it contains a wider range of phytochemicals and you are more likely to react to it. Note that cocoa and cacao can dry out the skin, whether you have amine sensitivity or not, so they are not a regular part of the programs in this book and consuming them on an ongoing basis may affect your results. If you have a worsening of symptoms, stop the test and let your skin recover — it is likely to be amine sensitivity or an allergy to a particular food. If you have not reacted so far, keep testing.

Day 20: If you are not sensitive or allergic to seafood, eat fresh salmon (not smoked or pickled) or pre-frozen white fish. Other amine-rich products you can test instead include dairy-free probiotics (plain, no dairy) or fish oils (no additives or flavourings, just pure oil). If you have a worsening of symptoms, stop the test and let your skin recover.

Day 21: Stop eating amine-rich foods for now (if there was no reaction you can eat them again after the salicylate test week). Prepare for the salicylate test and go shopping. If you reacted to the amine challenge wait until your symptoms subside before beginning the salicylate test.

> **Amine research**
>
> Amines can cause vasodilatation of the blood vessels, which can worsen topical steroid withdrawal (TSW), headaches and rosacea symptoms. Amine intolerance occurs in 36 per cent of people with eczema and 62 per cent of people who suffer from a range of systemic symptoms (affecting the whole body), including chronic fatigue, hay fever and asthma.[5]

Days 22 to 29: test salicylates

Continue to avoid eating amine-rich foods while you test salicylates. See if you react to salicylates with the following tests.

Days 22 to 23: Test medium-salicylate foods including carrots, snow peas (mangetout), butternut pumpkin (squash), mango and beetroot (beets).

Day 24: Test high amounts of flaxseed oil or flaxseeds/linseeds (also contains amines so you need to have passed the amine challenge). Children (over age 1) can have 1 teaspoon of flaxseed oil per day; teens and adults can have 2–3 teaspoons per day, with food. If you adversely reacted to amines last week, skip to Day 25.

Days 25 to 26: Test high-salicylate foods including capsicum (bell pepper), zucchini (courgette), cucumber, alfalfa, apricot, strawberries and/or blueberries. Enjoy!

Days 27 to 29: Test very high-salicylate foods including honey and curry powder or other spices *(but*

If you have an adverse reaction at any time, stop the salicylate challenge and take calcium carbonate powder (see www.eczemalife.com to order Skin Friend AM and PM) to speed up salicylate removal from the body.

avoid coconut milk and other non-listed ingredients). If there are no reactions within seven to ten days of beginning the salicylate challenge, then you are not sensitive to salicylates and you can continue eating these foods. If you are really unsure of the results, you can test aspirin as it has higher level of salicylates (do not test aspirin if you have asthma). If you adversely react to aspirin take a double dose of Skin Friend AM straight afterwards.

Days 30 to 36 : test MSG/glutamates

If you pass both the salicylate and amine challenges, then test MSG/glutamates.

Days 30 to 33: Test soy sauce (contains MSG/glutamates and amines), or test supplements that you would like to consume such as glutamine powder (Musashi) or pure pea protein powder (no other ingredients or flavourings) as they both contain glutamates. If you have no adverse reactions go to Day 34.

Day 34: Test pure MSG powder (caution: not if you have asthma). It's available via Amazon, selected Asian grocery stores and online. Why buy pure MSG? It's often useful to test the pure nutrient so if you react you know it's MSG sensitivity, not a food allergy.

Day 35: Test raw unsalted cashew nuts if you are not allergic to nuts. This is an optional test, as cashews are low-salicylate and a part of the Eczema Detox Program so it helps to know if you are sensitive to them or not.

Day 36: Test eggs if you would like to eat eggs. This is an optional test as quality free range or organic eggs can be added to the Eczema Detox Program if you are absolutely sure they don't trigger any type of adverse reaction.

Salicylate research

Salicylate intolerance occurs in 52 per cent of people with eczema, 62 per cent of people with hives, 69 per cent of people with IBS, 62 per cent of people with migraines, and 74 per cent of people with behavoural issues such as ADHD.[6]

Problem solving

If your skin worsens at all while on the elimination diet and you are unsure if salicylate or amines were involved, refer to Chapter 12, 'FAQs and problem solving'.

The Complete Salicylate Food Charts detail all foods from highest to lowest — to download a copy of the charts, see my website: www.eczemalife.com. Also refer to 'How to manage amine intolerance' on pp.118–9.

Case study: Charlie

You might have read how quickly this diet can work for some people and then be disheartened if it does not work as fast for you. While it can clear up eczema within one to twelve weeks, here is another case study highlighting how it can take longer to find your unique combination of trigger foods. Charlie shows it pays to be persistent ...

Charlie had eczema from birth to the age of twenty, when her condition improved. However, her eczema returned a couple of years later, triggered by an allergy to soy. Avoiding soy slightly improved her eczema but it had become severe and now the eczema covered most of her body.

Charlie said, 'I first started on The Eczema Diet book version and I noticed a small improvement within a month. When I did the stricter version (the Food Intolerance Diagnosis Program) and started taking Skin Friend AM and PM I noticed further improvements within a couple of weeks. I've been on the program for eight months now and I am still testing foods. Before I had eczema crusts on my whole body and now the crusts are only on my feet — they are still red but no longer swollen. I notice if I have a flare-up that I recover faster.'

Charlie is vegan and has salicylate sensitivity and adversely reacts to banana, potatoes and soy, and this limits her food options so she consumes pea protein powder for extra protein. As she still had eczema after eight months, I suspected she might also be sensitive to grains so I advised her to do a rotation diet to see if grains were affecting her eczema. The first week she avoided rice then reintroduced it and found she had a mild adverse reaction to basmati rice (contains salicylates) but not regular rice. Then she tested rye and had a severe reaction. So she now avoids both ingredients. Note these foods did not show up on allergy tests but they visibly worsened her skin during the elimination diet — this is why real-life diet challenges can be useful. Charlie suspects she reacts to buckwheat so she is now testing it by avoiding buckwheat for five days, then she will eat it and see if her skin worsens. She can successfully eat spelt without adverse reactions, so gluten, starch and grains (in general) are not a problem. Since identifying her trigger foods Charlie's skin has mostly cleared up, with the exception of her feet, which are slowly healing.

Chapter 9
Eczema Detox Program and menus

This chapter will give you all the information you need to follow the Eczema Detox Program. If you have already completed the FID Program you should have a good idea what your trigger foods are. If you are unsure, you can still begin here and see how your skin responds. The goal of this particular program is to be healthy and enjoy the delicious recipes.

Low- to medium-salicylate foods

You'll note the Eczema Detox Program allows both low-salicylate and medium-salicylate foods, as it is a less restrictive program than the FID Program.

The Eczema Detox food shopping list on p. 92 outlines the foods you can eat when following the Eczema Detox Program. The list includes food chemical abbreviations such as (S) which indicates the food or beverage contains salicylates. Other symbols indicate a food contains amines (A), glutamates/MSG (M), gluten (G), nitrates (N), tannins (T), goitrogens (O) and lactose (L). So if you know your chemical 'triggers' you can avoid these foods if needed. If you know you adversely react to items such as beans or fructose (etc.), you can continue to avoid these ingredients too.

What to eat daily (important!)

The following is a guide to the number of servings from the various food groups you should aim to eat each day for good health and satiety:

- » 2 x quality protein foods (lean meats, small white fish, legumes)
- » 1–2 x quality carbohydrates (rice, quinoa, buckwheat, peeled potato, etc.)
- » 5+ low- to medium-salicylate vegetables (refer to food list on pp. 92–3).
- » 1–2 x low- to medium-salicylate fruits (peeled to reduce salicylate content).
- » 1 x omega-3 rich food. Choose from: fish, flaxseeds/linseeds and/or chia seeds (whichever source you don't adversely react to). Note: fresh white fish or salmon are good options if you are not sensitive or allergic to seafood
- » 1 x purple food (cooked red cabbage, black beans or beetroot/beets)
- » 1–2 x orange foods (carrots, sweet potato or papaya/pawpaw)
- » 1–2 x green vegetables (lettuce, green beans, parsley, chives, spring onions/shallots/scallions etc.).

Frozen fruit

Keep a constant small supply of frozen banana, papaya or pawpaw (not other fruits) for making chilled smoothies and dairy-free Nice Cream, which is a lovely ice-cream alternative. Peel and chop the fruit and place the pieces into sealable freezer bags or containers and store in the freezer.

Note: frozen banana will go brown within three days so use it up quickly.

The menus

Note there are two sample menus to choose from: one for vegetarians and vegans, and a second menu for meat-eaters. For children, 'non-cooks' and picky eaters, refer to the children's FID menus on p. 98–9.

Eczema Detox Program: 7-day **vegan/vegetarian** menu

Here are some meal ideas that are rich in vegetarian protein and alkalizing ingredients for healthy skin. If you like juicing, add the juice recipes to your daily meals (see 'Snacks' opposite). Feel free to choose other recipes in this book to suit your allergies and preferences. Ensure you consume enough protein, omega-3 and alkalizing vegetables daily.

	Breakfast	Lunch	Dinner
Day 1	Protein Smoothie Bowl (p. 194) or Healthy Skin Smoothie with protein powder (p. 185) ½ to 2 teaspoons flaxseed oil	Lentil Vegie Soup (p. 164) or Alkaline Bomb Salad (p. 153) with Maple Dressing (p. 135)	Lentil Vegie Soup (p. 164) or Roasted Sweet Potato Salad (p. 202)
Day 2	Quinoa Porridge (p. 144) and/or Healthy Skin Smoothie with protein powder (p. 185) ½ to 2 teaspoons flaxseed oil	Lentil Vegie Soup (p. 164) or Alkaline Bomb Salad (p. 153) with Maple Dressing (p. 135)	Pumpkin and Snow Pea Bowl (p. 197) (optional white rice) and Healthy Skin Juice (p. 187)
Day 3	Wholegrain Oat Porridge (p. 142) or Healthy Skin Smoothie with protein powder (p. 185) ½ to 2 teaspoons flaxseed oil	Lentil Patties (p. 160) in Spelt Flat Bread (p. 155) and salad or Healthy Skin Smoothie with protein powder (p. 185)	Lentil Patties (p. 160) or Lentil Sausage Rolls (p.200) with cooked white rice, carrots and green beans, or Potato and Pesto Pizza (p. 156)
Day 4	Pumpkin and Snow Pea Bowl (p. 197) or Potato and Leek Waffles (p. 147), and Celery Cleansing Juice (p. 125) ½ to 2 teaspoons flaxseed oil	Mung Bean Sprout Pancakes (p. 168) and Healthy Skin Smoothie with protein powder (p. 185)	Papaya Rice Paper Rolls (with tofu) (p. 208) or leftovers (freeze banana or papaya for tomorrow's Nice Cream dessert; and save three ripe bananas for Banana Bread)
Day 5	Beans on Toast (p. 138) or easy option: plain puffed rice cereal and rice milk with peeled pear ½ to 2 teaspoons flaxseed oil	Herbed Tofu Open Sandwich (p. 159) or Design-your-own Sandwich (p. 158)	Wombok Noodle Salad with tofu (vegan option; p. 175) or leftovers, and Banana Nice Cream (p. 216) or Papaya Nice Cream (p. 216)

	Breakfast	Lunch	Dinner
Day 6	Potato and Leek Waffles (p. 147) and Celery Cleansing Juice (p. 125) or Sprout Smoothie (p. 187) ½ to 2 teaspoons flaxseed oil	Protein Smoothie Bowl (p. 194) or Healthy Skin Smoothie with protein powder (p. 185)	Simple San Choy Bau (p. 210) or San Choy Bau (vegan option; p. 171) and Banana Bread (p. 212)
Day 7	Banana Bread (p, 212) or Raw Omega Muesli (p. 193) and Healthy Skin Smoothie (p. 185) ½ to 2 teaspoons flaxseed oil	Leftover San Choy Bau or Healthy Skin Smoothie (p. 185)	Potato and Pesto Pizza (p. 156) with Caramelized Leek Sauce (p. 130), or Lentil Patties (p. 160) with Tasty Antioxidant Coleslaw (p. 202)

Snacks: The Wishing Plate (p. 148); Sesame-free Hummus (p. 132); Bean Dip (p. 132); Parsley Pesto (p. 189) with plain rice crackers; Banana Bread (p. 212) with Pink Pear Jam (p. 137).

Drinks: 1–3 litres filtered water; Pear and Vanilla Tea (p. 126); Healthy Skin Smoothie (p. 185) with 2 tablespoons pea/rice protein powder; Celery Cleansing Juice (p. 125); Healthy Skin Juice (p. 187); Alkaline Vegetable Broth (p. 167); Carob Tea (p. 126); Saffron Tea (p. 128); Electrolyte Pear Juice (p. 128).

Desserts: Carob Chia Pudding (p. 215); Banana Bread (p. 212); Spelt Pancakes (p. 141); Banana Buckwheat Pancakes (p. 190); Pear Spelt Muffins (p. 151); Pear Crumble (p. 178); Pear Sorbet (p. 181; or an iceblock/ice lolly/popsicle); Banana Nice Cream (p. 216); Papaya Nice Cream (p. 216).

Choose from any recipe in this book. Note there are many gluten-free options.

7-day Eczema Detox Program menu (for meat eaters)

Choose any meal in any order you like. Ensure you have protein twice a day and drink 1–3 litres of filtered water to help the detoxification process. Juicing is your liver's best friend, so remember to have homemade juices at least three times a week. Make Lentil Vegie Soup the day before you begin (or choose another meal). Enjoy!

	Breakfast	Lunch	Dinner
Day 1	Banana Beet Smoothie Bowl (p. 193) or Pumpkin and Snow Pea Bowl (p. 197) ½ to 2 teaspoons flaxseed oil	Lentil Vegie Soup (p. 164) or Alkaline Bomb Salad (p. 153) with Maple Dressing (p. 135)	Steamed Salmon with Maple Dressing, served with rice (p. 204), or Lentil Vegie Soup (p. 164)
Day 2	Quinoa Porridge (p. 144) or Wholegrain Oat Porridge (p. 142) and Healthy Skin Juice (p. 187) ½ to 2 teaspoons flaxseed oil	Leftover soup or Design-your-own Sandwich (p. 158)	Wombok Noodle Salad with chicken (p. 175) and Maple Dressing (p. 135)
Day 3	Pumpkin and Snow Pea Bowl (p. 197) or Healthy Skin Smoothie (p. 185) ½ to 2 teaspoons flaxseed oil	Alkaline Bomb Salad (p. 153; you can serve it with skinless chicken if desired)	Simple San Choy Bau (p. 210) or San Choy Bau (p. 171) (make Spelt Flat Bread, p. 155, for tomorrow's lunch)
Day 4	Wholegrain Oat Porridge (p. 142) or Banana Beet Smoothie Bowl (p. 193), Healthy Skin Juice (p. 187) ½ to 2 teaspoons flaxseed oil	Design-your-own Sandwich (p. 158) or Lentil Patties (p. 160) wrapped in Spelt Flat Bread (p. 155) with salad	Crispy Chicken Pasta (p. 176) (freeze banana or papaya for tomorrow's Nice Cream dessert)
Day 5	Beans on Toast (p. 138) or easy option: plain puffed rice cereal and rice milk with sliced papaya), Celery Cleansing Juice (p. 125) ½ to 2 teaspoons flaxseed oil	Mung Bean Sprout Pancakes (p. 168) or Design-your-own Sandwich (p. 158)	Potato and Pesto Pizza (p. 156) with Caramelized Leek Sauce (p. 130), Banana Nice Cream (p. 216)
Day 6	Banana Beet Smoothie Bowl (p. 193) ½ to 2 teaspoons flaxseed oil	Potato and Pesto Pizza (p. 156), or Design-your-own Sandwich (p. 158)	Steamed Fish Parcels with Mashed Potato (p. 172) or Sweet Potato Soup (p. 203) or Salmon Besan Pie (p. 207)

	Breakfast	Lunch	Dinner
Day 7	Potato and Leek Waffles (p. 147), Healthy Skin Juice (p. 187) ½ to 2 teaspoons flaxseed oil	Sweet Potato Soup (p. 203) or Protein Vegie Bowl (p. 140)	Sweet Potato Soup (p. 203) or Tasty Antioxidant Coleslaw (p. 202) with meat of choice

Snacks, drinks and desserts: See the snacks, drinks and desserts listed on p. 89)

Special occasions, birthdays etc.: See 'Eczema-friendly party treats' on p. 79.

Note: if you have any problems along the way, refer to Chapter 12, 'FAQs and problem solving' or join our Eczema Diet support group (see 'Useful resources' for details on p. 220).

	LOW SALICYLATES	MEDIUM SALICYLATES (do not eat all foods in this column at once – start with small amounts)
FRUIT	☐ peeled pears [T] ☐ bananas (*not sugar/ladyfinger*) [A, T] ☐ pawpaw [A] ☐ papaya [A]	☐ golden delicious apples [S, T] ☐ red delicious apples [S, T] [*strictly no other apples*] ☐ mango [S, T]
VEGETABLES	☐ Brussels sprouts [O] ☐ red cabbage [O, T] ☐ white cabbage [O] ☐ celery [N] ☐ dried beans ☐ dried peas (*not fresh or frozen*) ☐ green beans ☐ iceberg lettuce ☐ leeks ☐ mung bean sprouts ☐ white potato (e.g. Coliban, Kennebec, Sebago, brushed) ☐ shallots (spring onions/scallions) ☐ swede (rutabaga) ☐ yellow split peas (dried only)	☐ asparagus [S] ☐ beetroot (beets) [S] ☐ bok choy [S] ☐ carrot [S] ☐ cos (romaine) lettuce [S] ☐ parsnips [S] ☐ low GI potatoes (new, Carisma*; S) ☐ pumpkin (winter squash) [S, T] ☐ snow peas (mangetout) [S] ☐ bean sprouts [S] ☐ sweet potato [S] ☐ turnip [S] *salicylate content unknown
HERBS + SPICES	☐ chives, fresh/dried ☐ garlic, fresh ☐ parsley, fresh/dried ☐ garlic powder ☐ saffron	
VEGAN PROTEIN	☐ beans (most types but *not broad beans/fava beans*) ☐ chickpeas (garbanzo beans) ☐ legumes ☐ lentils (red/brown etc.) ☐ poppy seeds ☐ pea protein powder (no flavouring) ☐ tofu (plain) ☐ cashews (raw only)	☐ chia seeds [S, A] ☐ flaxseeds/linseeds [S, A] ☐ flaxseed oil [S, A]
ANIMAL PROTEIN	Choose organic or free-range where possible: ☐ beef ☐ chicken (must be skinless) ☐ fish (white, small, fresh, flathead, hake, John dory etc.) ☐ lamb ☐ rabbit ☐ veal ☐ Caution: eggs (for baking)	High amines: ☐ salmon [A] ☐ trout [A] ☐ rainbow trout [A] All fish should be fresh (*avoid frozen, dried, pickled, salted or smoked fish*)

	LOW SALICYLATES	MEDIUM SALICYLATES (do not eat all foods in this column at once – start with small amounts)
CARBOHYDRATES: GRAINS, FLOURS, GLUTEN	Gluten-free: ☐ arrowroot ☐ buckwheat ☐ gluten-free oats ☐ gluten-free rice pasta ☐ Doongara low GI rice (Sunrice Clever Rice) ☐ brown rice ☐ sushi rice (do not add vinegar) ☐ white rice (avoid jasmine and basmati rice) ☐ plain rice cereal (puffed, plain) ☐ white quinoa, quinoa flakes ☐ rice noodles (plain) ☐ sago ☐ millet Contains gluten: barley (G) ☐ oats (plain; G) ☐ rolled oats (G) ☐ rye (G) ☐ wheat-free sourdough spelt bread (S) ☐ spelt flour (G)	☐ psyllium* ☐ red quinoa* *may contain salicylates (content unknown)
BEVERAGES	☐ organic soy milk (if not allergic, plain, no seaweed or flavours) ☐ rice milk (plain) ☐ mineral water (plain, no colours or flavouring) ☐ spring water ☐ oat milk	
SWEETENERS + FLAVOURINGS	☐ carob powder (*pref. not roasted;* T) ☐ maple syrup (pure/real) ☐ Carob Syrup (T) (see p. 134) ☐ carob nibs (T) see 'Useful resources' p. 221 ☐ rice malt syrup (brown rice syrup) ☐ quality sea salt (*no anti-caking agent*) ☐ vanilla (T) (real, *not imitation*)	
OILS + FATS	☐ rice bran oil* or brown rice oil If you are allergic to rice, try safflower oil or sunflower oil (*avoid antioxidant 320/BHA*)	☐ flaxseed oil (S, A) (small bottle or capsules, must be unflavoured)
SNACK FOODS	☐ raw unsalted cashews ☐ celery ☐ plain rice cakes (*no flavourings*) ☐ plain rice crackers (e.g. Sakata plain rice crackers or Peckish Brown Rice Crackers 'no salt' variety only)	☐ carrots

As this diet permits time off for social events, refer to p. 79 for eczema-friendly party treats. If you have a day off, simply return to the Eczema Detox Program the next day. You do not have to eat everything on this list. Note: cashews are not suitable for people with a nut allergy.

Chapter 10
FID Program menus and children's menus

This chapter outlines Food Intolerance Diagnosis (FID) menu plans for children, novice cooks, non-cooks, people with gluten intolerance and fussy eaters. The first menu utilizes easy-to-make low-salicylate recipes and store-bought ingredients for the FID Program. Follow this menu first (or one of the other week 1–2 menus) then progress to the 'Amine test menu', (week 3) and the 'Salicylate test menu' (week 4) to test and enjoy a wider range of foods. If you have any adverse reactions during weeks 3 to 4 then revert to one of the week 1–2 menus in this chapter and read the advice in the FID Program chapter (see p. 76).

Tips for success

The FID Program needs to be followed strictly for two weeks (followed by two weeks of testing) in order to accurately diagnose chemical sensitivities. The good news is after you have completed this testing phase you can have days off and special meals.

Here are some tips for success:

» There is a limit of two peeled pears per day during the FID Program.

» Fresh pears should be ripe and peeled. Avoid Nashi (Asian) and Ya pears and any pears that are hard or apple-shaped, as they contain salicylates.

» Consume a very small amount of flaxseed oil to receive your daily intake of omega-3. Teens and adults should have ½ teaspoon daily (but not more for the first two weeks; you can test larger amounts in week 3). See the children's menu (pp. 98–9) for the child dose.

» Photocopy the FID shopping list on p. 78 so you can take it with you when shopping.

» Take a photo of your (or your child's) eczema before you begin, and again each month, so you can monitor progress. It's easy to forget how bad your skin was before you began!

» Buy a new waffle iron — it will be your new best friend as the waffle recipes are easy to make and there are delicious varieties to suit all tastes.

What to eat daily

The following is a guide to the number of servings from the various food groups you should aim to eat each day for good health and satiety:

» 2 x quality protein foods (lean meats, small white fish, legumes)

» 3 x quality carbohydrates (rice, quinoa, buckwheat, peeled potato, etc.)

» 5+ low-salicylate vegetables (refer to food lists on pp. 92–3).

» 1–2 x low-salicylate fruits (fruits must be peeled to reduce salicylate content)

» 1 x omega-3 rich food. Choose from: fish and/or flaxseeds/linseeds (whichever source you don't adversely react to).

» 1 x purple food eaten four times per week (cooked red cabbage or black beans)

» 3 x green vegetables (mung bean sprouts, lettuce, green beans, parsley, chives, spring onions/shallots/scallions)

» 1 x anti-inflammatory vegetable (leek, spring onions/shallots/scallions or garlic)

How much protein per serving?

If eating meat, have a protein serving the size of the palm of your hand. If serving to a child, then a child-sized palm is your reference. While daily protein consumption is very important for healthy skin, animal protein foods are not to be overeaten. You can eat animal protein twice a day, including omega-3 rich fish two to three times *per week*. Vegan protein can be eaten in larger amounts. If you are vegetarian or vegan, have an additional 2–3 tablespoons of pea/rice protein powder daily so you consume enough quality protein for healthy skin (refer to p. 29 for details).

Easy FID menu (for weeks 1–2)

The following is an example of a 7-day menu that can be used during the 14-day elimination diet and whenever you need it. This menu includes fast and easy recipes. Other options include the children's menu (pp. 98–9), infant's program (for babies under age one, pp. 108–9) and the gluten-free menu (pp. 100–1). Further instructions can be found in Chapter 8, 'Food Intolerance Diagnosis (FID) Program'.

Note there is a lot of food on the following menus and you don't have to eat everything on the menu. You can also change the order of the recipes to use up leftovers (but *do not eat leftover meats during the two-week elimination period as they develop amines overnight —* you can have them in week 3).

7-day easy FID menu (for weeks 1–2)

This menu is ideal for non-cooks, novice cooks, children and fussy eaters. Vegan/vegetarian meal options are included.

	Breakfast	Snacks/lunchbox	Lunch	Dinner/dessert
Day 1	plain puffed rice cereal and calcium-fortified rice milk	fresh peeled pear or canned pear (syrup drained), plain rice crackers and/or celery sticks with Sesame-free Hummus (p. 132)	Oat Waffles (p. 145)	Crispy Chicken Pasta (p. 176) or Lentil Vegie Soup (p. 164)
Day 2	Wholegrain Oat Porridge (p. 142) or Carob Milkshake (p. 129)	fresh peeled pear or canned pear (drained), large rice cakes with Sesame-free Hummus (p. 132)	Design-your-own Sandwich (p. 158) (FID options: avoid salicylate foods such as carrot)	Lentil Vegie Soup (no carrot, p. 164) (freeze canned or stewed pears for tomorrow night's Pear Sorbet, p. 181)
Day 3	Protein Vegie Bowl (p. 140)	plain rice crackers (plain salted) with Bean Dip (p. 132)	Design-your-own Sandwich (p. 158) (choose FID options)	Simple San Choy Bau with optional rice (p. 210) Pear Sorbet (p. 181)

	Breakfast	Snacks/lunchbox	Lunch	Dinner/dessert
Day 4	plain puffed rice cereal and rice milk	celery sticks, fresh peeled pear, plain rice crackers (plain salted) with Bean Dip (p. 132)	Design-your-own Sandwich (p. 158) (choose FID options)	Protein Vegie Bowl (p. 140)
Day 5	Beans on Toast (p. 138)	fresh peeled pear, plain wholegrain rice crackers with Bean Dip (p. 132)	Design-your-own Sandwich (p. 158)	Crispy Chicken Pasta (p. 176) or New Potato and Leek Soup (p. 163)
Day 6	plain puffed rice cereal and rice milk	fresh peeled pear, celery sticks and plain wholegrain rice crackers with Bean Dip (p. 132)	Design-your-own Sandwich (low-salicylate options, no nuts or banana, p. 158)	Steamed Fish Parcels with Mashed Potato (p. 172) or leftover New Potato and Leek Soup (p. 163) (optional: freeze canned pears for tomorrow night's Pear Sorbet, p. 181)
Day 7	Wholegrain Oat Porridge (p. 142)	fresh peeled pear or leftovers, plain rice crackers and Sesame-free Hummus (p. 132) or Bean Dip (p. 132)	one of the waffle recipes or Protein Vegie Bowl (p. 140)	Lamb and Sticky Leeks (p. 170) or Mung Bean Sprout Pancakes (p. 168) with Sesame-free Hummus (p. 132) Pear Sorbet (p. 181)

If you are sensitive to any item on the menu, avoid it and use a substitute from the FID food shopping list (p. 78).

Drinks: filtered or spring water (no flavourings); pure mineral water (no flavouring); Carob Tea (p. 126); Saffron Tea (p. 128); Pear and Vanilla Tea (p. 126); Carob Milkshake (p. 129); Celery Cleansing Juice (p. 125); Electrolyte Pear Juice (p. 128); calcium-fortified rice milk.

Children's FID menu (for weeks 1–2)

This menu includes lunchbox items and easy meals for fussy eaters and the whole family. It is often easier to cook the same recipe for the whole family.

Here are some tips for following the children's FID menu:

» Use up your leftovers and be creative! Adjust the portion sizes to suit your child's age and feeding ability.
» Peeled fresh pear goes brown quickly in lunchboxes so it's better to make stewed pear or pack canned pear pieces (sugar syrup, drained).
» Make the Pink Pear Jam (p. 137) and Sesame-free Hummus (p. 132) in advance.
» I highly recommend the Potato and Leek Waffles (p. 147) and Pear Crumble (p. 178).
» Also refer to the tips at the beginning of this chapter.

7-day children's FID menu (for weeks 1–2)

Some recipes contain gluten, so refer to the gluten-free menu if needed. Meals are suggestions only and not every meal has to be eaten.

	Breakfast	Snacks/lunchbox	Lunch	Dinner/dessert
Day 1	spelt sourdough toast with Pink Pear Jam (p. 137) or puffed rice cereal and calcium-fortified rice milk	canned pear (drained), Pear Spelt Muffins (p. 151), plain rice crackers and/or celery sticks with Sesame-free Hummus (p. 132)	Potato and Leek Waffles (p. 147) or Oat Waffles (p. 145)	Crispy Chicken Pasta (p. 176) Pear Crumble (p. 178) or Carob Milkshake (p. 129)
Day 2	Wholegrain Oat Porridge (p. 142)	canned pear (drained), Pear Spelt Muffins (p. 151), large rice cakes with Sesame-free Hummus (p. 132)	Design-your-own Sandwich (p. 158) (add chicken and avoid salicylate foods such as carrot)	Lentil Sausage Rolls (p. 200) (beef or lamb option, if desired), lemonade iceblock (ice lolly/popsicle, store-bought, no colourings) or warm rice milk
Day 3	plain puffed rice cereal and rice milk with sliced pear (peeled) or Protein Vegie Bowl (p. 140)	Pear Crumble (p. 178) or fresh peeled pear, plain rice crackers or rice cakes (plain salted)	Spelt Flat Bread (p. 155) with Crispy Chicken (see pasta recipe, p. 176) (optional: iceberg lettuce; chicken must be cooked today)	cooked organic mince with pasta and green beans or celery (avoid mince with preservatives) leftover Pear Crumble

	Breakfast	Snacks/lunchbox	Lunch	Dinner/dessert
Day 4	Oat Waffles (p. 145), with Pink Pear Jam (p. 137)	celery sticks (peeled to remove strings), leftover Pear Crumble or fresh peeled pear, plain rice crackers (plain salted)	Design-your-own Sandwich (p. 158)	Steamed Fish Parcels with Mashed Potato (p. 172), Carob Milkshake (p. 129)
Day 5	Beans on Toast (p. 138)	fresh peeled pear or Pear Crumble (p. 178), plain wholegrain rice crackers with Bean Dip (p. 132)	Design-your-own Sandwich (p. 158)	Lentil Vegie Soup (no carrot; p. 164), lemonade iceblock (ice lolly/popsicle) or 1 cup warm calcium-fortified rice milk (make New Anzac Cookies (p. 182) for tomorrow)
Day 6	plain puffed rice cereal and rice milk	fresh peeled pear or canned pear (sugar syrup drained), New Anzac Cookies (p. 182) The Wishing Plate (p. 148) with celery and Sesame-free Hummus (p. 132)	Design-your-own Sandwich (p. 158) (low-salicylate options, no nuts or banana,)	Lamb and Sticky Leeks (p. 170) (optional: freeze canned or stewed pears for Pear Sorbet (p. 181) tomorrow night)
Day 7	Wholegrain Oat Porridge (p. 142)	fresh peeled pear or Pear Crumble leftovers, New Anzac Cookies (p. 182), plain rice crackers and Sesame-free Hummus (p. 132)	Potato and Leek Waffles (p. 147) with Sesame-free Hummus (p. 132)	Simple San Choy Bau (p. 210) or Lentil Vegie Soup (p. 164) Pear Sorbet (p. 181)

If you are sensitive to any item on the menu, avoid it and use a substitute from the FID food shopping list (p. 78). Refer to the drinks menu on p. 97.

Gluten-free FID menu (for weeks 1–2)

If you would like to (or need to) eat gluten-free, this menu will help you to choose the right meals. If you are unsure if you adversely react to gluten, you can follow this menu for two weeks, then from days 15–20 eat foods containing gluten. Try spelt, rye and oats and see if your eczema worsens or if any other adverse symptom appears. If there are no adverse reactions within one to ten days you are not gluten intolerant. Note: do not test other foods during this test period as your results may be unclear.

To prepare for breakfast on Day 1, make Carob Chia Pudding (p. 215), using sago instead of chia — it needs time to set.

7-day Gluten-free FID menu (for weeks 1–2)

Remember to use up leftovers, with the exception of leftover meats which should be avoided, as they develop amines when stored overnight after cooking.

	Breakfast	Snacks/lunchbox	Lunch	Dinner/dessert
Day 1	Carob Chia Pudding (use sago instead of chia; p. 215)	fresh peeled pear, plain rice crackers (plain salted, no additives), and/or celery sticks (peeled to remove strings) with Sesame-free Hummus (p. 132)	Potato and Leek Waffles (p. 147) with optional Sesame-free Hummus (p. 132)	Wombok Noodle Salad, gluten-free option (p. 175)
Day 2	Protein Vegie Bowl (p. 140)	fresh peeled pear or canned pear (sugar syrup, drained), large rice cakes and peeled celery sticks with Sesame-free Hummus (p. 132)	Design-your-own Sandwich (p. 158) (avoid gluten and salicylate foods such as carrot)	Lentil Vegie Soup (no carrot; p. 164) (make Pear Crumble, gluten-free version, for tomorrow's snack, p. 178)
Day 3	Wholegrain Oat Porridge (gluten-free oats) (p. 142) or Potato and Leek Waffles (p. 147) with Sesame-free Hummus (p. 132)	Pear Crumble (p. 178) using GF oats and GF quinoa flakes, or fresh peeled pear, plain rice crackers (plain salted)	Lentil Vegie Soup leftovers	San Choy Bau (p. 171) or Simple San Choy Bau (p. 210)

	Breakfast	Snacks/lunchbox	Lunch	Dinner/dessert
Day 4	Protein Vegie Bowl (p. 140)	celery sticks (peeled to remove strings); Celery Cleansing Juice (p. 125), leftover Pear Crumble or fresh peeled pear, plain rice crackers (plain salted)	Alkaline Bomb Salad (p. 153)	Steamed Fish Parcels with Mashed Potato (p. 172)
Day 5	Quinoa Porridge (p. 144) Carob Tea (p. 126)	fresh peeled pear or canned pear (syrup drained), plain rice crackers (plain salted), celery sticks with Bean Dip (p. 132)	Design-your-own Sandwich (p. 158)	Lamb and Sticky Leeks (p. 170)
Day 6	Mung Bean Sprout Pancakes (p. 168)	Pear Crumble leftovers Celery Cleansing Juice (p.125)	Protein Vegie Bowl (p. 140)	Crispy Chicken Pasta (p. 176)
Day 7	Quinoa Porridge (p. 144), or Beans on Toast (with no toast, p. 138)	plain rice crackers and Sesame-free Hummus (p. 132) celery sticks (peeled to remove strings)	Protein Vegie Bowl (p. 140) with chicken or lamb	New Potato and Leek Soup (p. 163)

If you are sensitive to any item on the menu, avoid it and use a substitute from the FID shopping list (p. 78). Refer to the drinks menu on p. 97.

Drinks: 1–3 litres of filtered or natural spring water; Pear and Vanilla Tea (p. 126); Celery Cleansing Juice (p. 125); Alkaline Vegetable Broth (p. 167); Carob Tea. (p. 126); Saffron Tea (p. 128); Electrolyte Pear Juice (p. 128); plain mineral water.

Desserts: Pear Sorbet (p. 181); Carob Milkshake (p. 129); Oat Waffles (p. 145, using gluten-free oats) with Pink Pear Jam (p. 137); Pear Crumble (gluten-free option; p. 178).

Additives to avoid

In the bid to prevent eczema it's important to avoid itch-promoting additives when you buy packaged or fresh foods. Use this table to look up additives to avoid.

Additive	Number/s	Food sources
flavour enhancers: glutamates, monosodium glutamate (MSG)	620–635	flavoured noodles, chicken-salted chips (crisps), flavoured crackers and crisps, sauces, stock cubes, gravies, fast foods, traditional Chinese cooking (natural sources of MSG include tomato, soy sauce, broccoli, mushrooms, spinach, grapes, plums, deli meats, miso, tempeh, wine, rum, sherry, brandy, liqueur)
artificial colourings: tartrazine (yellow), red, blue, green, black, brown	102, 104, 107, 110, 122–129, 132, 133, 142, 151, 155 (US: blue 1 and 2, green 3, red 2, 3, 4 and 40, yellow 5 and 6)	confectionery/lollies/candy, jelly (jello), breakfast cereals, glacé cherries, salmon, hot dogs (frankfurters), soft drinks, flavoured mineral water, chocolate, potato crisps, corn chips, toppings, ice-cream, iceblocks (popsicles/ice lollies), fruit drinks, cordials, flavoured milks, meat pies, cupcakes, cakes, liqueur, yoghurt and dairy snacks
natural colouring	160b (annatto)	in many yoghurts, butter, fish fingers, custard and commercial desserts (160a is a safe alternative)
preservatives	sorbates 200–203, benzoates 210–213, sulphites 220–228, nitrites 249–252, propionates 280–283	used in some processed fruits and vegetables, wines, beer, most soft drinks (sodas), diet drinks, cordials, juices, processed meats, sausages, dried fruit, processed deli meats (e.g. sausages, devon, ham, salami); 282 in some breads, buns and wraps
antioxidant preservatives	310–321	in oils, margarines, chips (crisps), fried snack foods, fast foods
artificial sweeteners: aspartame, saccharin	951, 954	ice-creams, NutraSweet®, Equal®, Sweet 'N Low®, diet and 'sugar-free' products, diet soft drinks (sodas), 'zero' soft drinks, cakes, biscuits (cookies), sweet pies, muffins

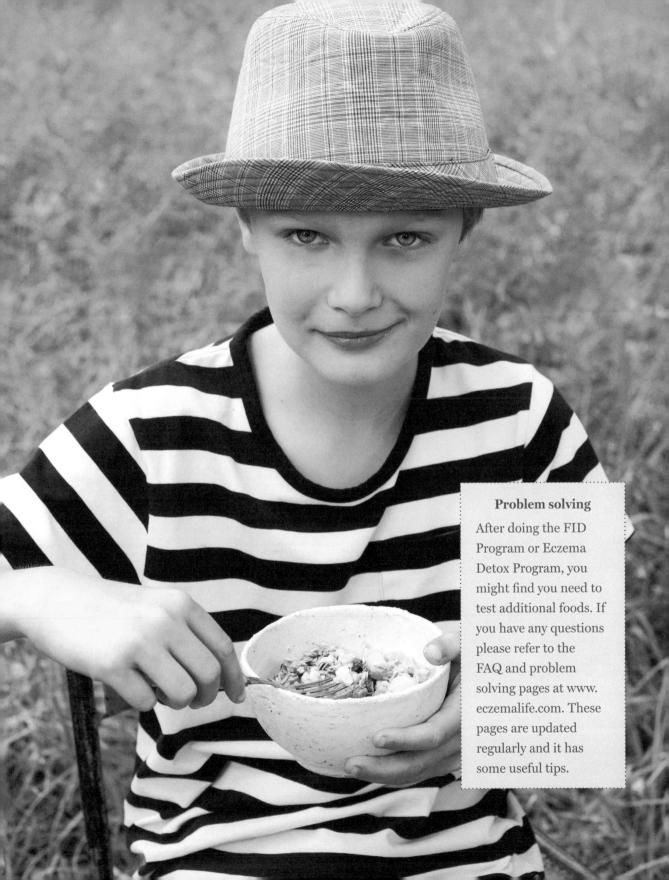

Problem solving

After doing the FID Program or Eczema Detox Program, you might find you need to test additional foods. If you have any questions please refer to the FAQ and problem solving pages at www. eczemalife.com. These pages are updated regularly and it has some useful tips.

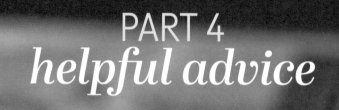

PART 4
helpful advice

Chapter 11
Babies with eczema

Babies can develop eczema before they reach the age of one, and it's important to avoid panicking if this occurs. As mentioned before, infants under the age of two naturally have under-functioning livers and this makes them prone to problems such as jaundice, cradle cap and eczema. It is perfectly normal for the liver to be unable to detoxify chemicals properly, which is why baby products usually contain fewer chemicals and are labelled 'hypoallergenic' (although many of these products are still loaded with chemicals!).

While your baby's only food source is milk (either breastmilk or formula), you have several ways to modify what types of nutrients he or she receives.

Breastfeeding tips

» When you are breastfeeding, the essential fatty acids, vitamins and minerals from your diet pass into your breastmilk, and your child's body uses these nutrients for growth, repair and maintenance.

» While you are breastfeeding, you can modify your own meals to be lower in natural plant chemicals and change the nutrient composition.

» You can avoid consuming the foods that are known to exacerbate eczema (see the 'Itchy Dozen worst foods for eczema' on p. 16).

» Alternatively, you can wait until your baby is older and on solid foods before beginning his or her treatment.

» You can also take skin supplements that are suitable for use during breastfeeding.

Note that babies are not to be directly given vitamin supplements (unless it is a suitable probiotic or prescribed), and breastfeeding mothers need their energy so ensure you are eating enough.

If you have a colicky or 'windy' baby, you might also need to avoid garlic, leeks and spring onions (shallots/scallions). Use the Eczema Detox food shopping list (the less restricted program), which is on pp. 92–3.

Infant formula

If your baby is drinking infant formula, speak to your paediatrician or doctor about changing your baby to a low-allergy, non-dairy formula.

Starting solids

Recent research shows that delaying the introduction of solids for more than six months can *increase* the risk of allergy and eczema so the current recommendation is to *start your baby on solids after four months of age*, unless advised otherwise by your paediatrician or doctor. This is a general recommendation and may not be suitable for all babies.

For example, your baby needs to be able to sit upright while eating and if your baby is not showing signs of being ready for solids you can delay introducing solids for up to six months.

Tips for starting solids

» 'One new food every three days ...' To identify allergies and intolerances, introduce each new food on its own and then continue with that food for three days before introducing the next food.

» It is a good idea to introduce new foods earlier in the day, rather than at bedtime, as once your baby is in bed you can't see if they are having an adverse reaction. If your child has swelling or difficulty in breathing, you can spot it early in the day and seek medical advice.

» When introducing a new food, if your baby has an adverse reaction such as a flare-up, unsettled behaviour, diarrhoea or vomiting, keep a record in a diet diary and discontinue use of that particular food. Diarrhoea and vomiting can cause dehydration so hydrating electrolytes may be required. Seek your doctor's advice if this occurs. A natural diarrhoea remedy for children who have started solids includes grated fresh pear mixed with a little carob powder.

» Avoid giving your baby foods they can choke on such as nuts, biscuits (cookies), toast and solid pieces of fruit or vegetables etc.

Intolerance awareness: If your child reacts to banana, papaya or pawpaw, he or she could be sensitive to amines. Pear is usually well tolerated but in rare cases of fructose or tannin intolerances, pear may cause reactions. Don't worry: pear is unlikely to cause any problems!

If your child reacts to mango, pumpkin (winter squash), carrot, apples or sweet potato they may be sensitive to salicylates. If this occurs, avoid these new foods for now and test them again in a couple of months' time.

Avoid fussy eaters: vegies first, fruit second

Don't give your baby fruit before vegetables, as they might develop a sweet tooth and reject savoury foods. It is essential that your baby consumes eczema-friendly vegetables on a daily basis, as vegetables are alkalizing and will help your child to be eczema-free.

Foods from twelve months onwards

Your child should be consuming chopped up foods by now to experience different textures and flavours. Refer to Chapter 10 for the children's menu.

Drinks

Best drinks for babies include breastmilk, non-dairy infant formula and pre-boiled and cooled water.

» For children under the age of one year, water must be filtered and then boiled to sterilize and kill bacteria, and then cooled before giving it to your baby.

» Do not give pre-boiled water to infants after the age of one, as your growing toddler's gastrointestinal tract needs to become accustomed to unsterilized water to challenge and strengthen their immune system.

» After the age of one, regular filtered water is recommended. Filtered tap water is okay if tap water is safe to drink in your country. In places such as Italy, quality bottled water is advised.

If you have a young child with eczema, give them foods that they are able to chew successfully. Adapt the recipes in this book to suit your baby — mash, puree etc.

Starting solids

Foods from 4 months	Foods from 6 months	Foods from 8 months
continue to feed your baby breastmilk or infant formula	breastmilk (or non-dairy infant formula)	breastmilk (or non-dairy infant formula)
plain baby rice cereal*: ensure it has added iron and choose plain varieties, no fruit flavours. If eczema symptoms worsen discontinue use and seek advice from a nutritionist. Quinoa may be a suitable alternative (but note it might not contain added iron).	iron-rich meat (one new food every 3 days)**: babies need extra iron in their diet for proper growth. When serving meat, ensure it is very finely ground and start with lean lamb and then try skinless chicken, both freshly minced, preservative-free, antibiotic-free, free range and/or organic if possible, and fresh not frozen (as leftovers develop amines).	if your baby is feeding well and ready for chunkier foods, you can give him or her small serves of the following: · soft eczema-friendly fruits · steamed carrot sticks · sweet potato · potato slices · steamed green beans.
pureed vegetables: eczema-safe vegetables are the best ones to try first. These include pureed white potato, sweet potato, carrot and choko (chayote) – all steamed and mashed.	continue to give your baby rice cereal, eczema-friendly vegetables and fruit, then add the following steamed and mashed veggies: · swede (rutabaga) · butternut pumpkin (butternut squash).	gluten-free rice or buckwheat pasta spirals (no corn/maize or wheat pastas, and no long spaghetti at this stage)
This is a time for investigation. Although reactions to these foods are rare, if your child reacts to sweet potato or carrot they could be sensitive to salicylates. If your child reacts to peeled white potato they could be sensitive to nightshades.	iron rich legumes: mushy lentils, mashed chickpeas (garbanzo beans), mashed kidney beans, dried split peas (boiled) and so on (but avoid broad beans as they are rich in salicylates and avoid fresh peas as they contain MSG and salicylates). Recipes: Lentil Vegie Soup (no added salt) (p. 164), Teething Rusks (p. 111)	

Foods from 4 months	Foods from 6 months	Foods from 8 months
pureed fruit: eczema-safe fruits are peeled pureed pear (not Nashi/Asian or Ya) (for variety, also see next column)	mashed banana (not sugar/lady finger variety), papaya and pawpaw.	mango (fresh only), stewed (peeled) red delicious or golden delicious apples (avoid other types as they are high in salicylates) Banana Nice Cream (p. 216)

*In rare instances babies can be allergic to rice or banana, so if your baby's eczema flares up within one to five days after eating these foods, discontinue use and find another nutritious food source, such as quinoa, with the guidance of a nutritionist.
**Do not give your baby liver or lamb's fry as liver is the organ that can accumulate pesticides and chemicals, and be too rich in vitamin A.

Foods to avoid

Avoid giving your baby potentially problematic foods such as dairy products (cheese, yoghurt, butter, cow's milk etc.), eggs, fish and peanut butter and other nuts and pastes including tahini/sesame seed paste. Speak to your doctor about allergy testing before your child consumes these foods. Fruit juice, cordial and soft drinks (sodas) are not recommended for babies.

Teething

If your baby is teething you can make homemade teething rusks that are wheat- and dairy-free. They're easy to make and the recipe is on p. 111.

Baby teething treatments

Baby teething gels often contain high salicylates that can cause eczema to worsen; plus they can damage the lining of the stomach. According to researchers, there are more effective teething treatments than salicylate-containing gels and these include children's paracetamol or ibuprofen for pain or fever, and cold teething rings.[1] Always check the label when using medications and do not exceed the daily recommended dose for your child's age and weight.

Recommendations

» Make your child as comfortable as possible and use their prescribed medicated creams, if desired.

» After your child turns one year old, read Chapter 10, 'FID Program menus and children's menus', which includes the children's menu and helpful tips.

Key points to remember

» Laugh and have fun with your eczema baby — laughter can help them to heal.

» Babies have naturally under-functioning livers so a low-chemical diet is a good way to start solids.

» Introduce one new food every three days so you can identify any problem foods early.

» Breastfeeding mothers can follow any of the programs in this book if you are not taking medications that prevent you from changing your diet. Ensure you are eating plenty of food and seek advice from a nutritionist.

» When your baby starts solids make meal times fun.

» If your child is a fussy eater, don't let them go hungry. Refer to my book *Healthy Family, Happy Family* to change their eating habits (see 'Useful resources' on pp. 220–1).

» If you need help, seek additional support via www.eczemalife.com and our support group (see 'Useful resources' on pp. 220–1).

Teething Rusks (gluten-free)

Makes 20+, cooking time 1–1½ hours

You can substitute the banana with 1 cup pureed stewed pear or any other eczema-safe fruit or vegetable, such as 1 cup cooked sweet potato (S), swede (rutabaga) or carrot (S). Ensure the rusks bake hard. Please note, when feeding your infant teething rusks, finger foods or any other food that could be a choking hazard, it's important to supervise your child and ensure they are sitting upright.

- 1 cup mashed banana
- 1 cup rice flour
- filtered water

Preheat the oven to 150°C (300°F). Using a food processor, puree the banana then add the flour and mix on low speed. Alternately, place the banana in a mixing bowl, mash with a fork and mix in the flour. Add water if necessary, *one teaspoon at a time*, to form a stiff, dry dough (do not make it wet).

On a floured chopping board, roll out the mixture into a long, thin sausage, then slice into pieces around 8 cm (3 in) long.

Line a baking tray with baking paper, place the rusks on the tray and place in the oven. Bake the rusks for 1–1½ hours or until they are hard (may take up to 2 hours, depending on how much liquid you have used). Store in an airtight container for up to a week.

Chapter 12
FAQs and problem solving

The following FAQs have been divided into general problem solving and food questions.

Food

'Leeks and garlic give me stomach cramps, so do I have to eat them?'

No, you don't have to eat them. Avoid foods that make you feel unwell.

'What are the best alkalizing foods to eat while following the programs?'

All of the vegetables are alkalizing, including potatoes, plus banana and rice malt syrup (brown rice syrup). If you are following the FID Program (the stricter program), the best *highly* alkalizing foods are mung bean sprouts, Brussels sprouts, cabbage, parsley, leeks and spring onions (shallots/ scallions, straight stem/no bulb). If you are following the Eczema Detox Program, eat highly alkalizing vegetables including beetroot (beets), lentil sprouts and bean sprouts, and the ones I just mentioned for the FID Program.

'I'm sensitive to pears and carob, so what can I eat as substitutes while following the FID Program?'

Pears and carob contain tannins so you might have tannin sensitivity. On the FID Program for the first two weeks it's important to avoid adding substitute fruits, but in week 3 you can test pawpaw, and if you are not sensitive to it, this is the best fruit for you to eat. If you pass the salicylate test you can eat some medium-salicylate fruits (see p. 92). However, if you are highly sensitive to tannin you might also react to salicylates so don't skip this test. Instead of carob, flavour your shakes with rice malt syrup or real maple syrup, or choose another recipe.

'I am sensitive to bananas and amines, so what can I put in my smoothies instead?'

Flavour your smoothies with carob powder, real vanilla, rice malt syrup or real maple syrup. To make your smoothies cold, pour rice milk (or a non-dairy milk from this book) into an ice cube tray and freeze it for use in smoothies.

'I did an allergy test and I'm not allergic to dairy, so can I eat dairy products during the program?'

Both the Eczema Detox and FID programs are dairy-free because avoiding dairy helps eczema to clear up faster, whether you have dairy allergy or not. Research shows that allergy testing is often inaccurate so it cannot be relied on for a proper diagnosis. For example, researchers tested

183 people with eczema using a variety of testing methods on the same group of people. They found 67 per cent of them adversely reacted to dairy during a *skin prick test*, yet the patch test tended to be negative immediately afterwards. Interestingly, the dairy patch test later became positive in 89 per cent of eczema sufferers who showed a *delayed* adverse reaction to dairy.[1] So if this group had relied on the skin prick test alone, 22 per cent of them would have falsely believed they were not allergic to dairy.

The Food Intolerance Diagnosis Program in this book will help you accurately diagnose intolerances and allergies and *once your eczema clears up* you can use the same diagnostic methods to test dairy products (see 'Additional tests' on p. 115 for instructions).

'I've heard coconut oil is good for eczema. Why is it not a part of your program?'

Coconut has become one of the most popular health food products of the decade but it's not good for eczema *if you are sensitive to salicylates or amines.* As coconut can aggravate eczema, it is not an ingredient used in this book. *While not everyone will adversely react to coconut, it contains very high levels of both salicylates and amines, which can promote the itch, and it is 99 per cent saturated fat, which is pro-inflammatory.* Adverse reactions can occur anywhere from three to seven days after consuming coconut, so it may be hard to identify coconut as a trigger food. The best way to tell is to avoid all coconut products during the program and, if you wish, test coconut once your eczema has cleared up.

'Is avocado good for eczema?'

I know the blogs tell you to eat avocado for eczema but if you are sensitive to salicylates or amines then avocado will make your skin itchy. It is one of the 'Itchy dozen worst foods for eczema' (see p. 116) so while your skin is flared up, avoid it. The Supplement Program in this book will help to eventually prevent adverse reactions to salicylates and amines. So once your eczema has healed and you want to eat avocado, test it for a few days and see if you react to it.

'Fructose and beans give me gas, so do I have to eat these ingredients while following the program?'

No. You don't have to. If you would like to try a recipe but you are sensitive to a particular ingredient, you can swap the ingredient using the FID food shopping list as a guide (see p. 78). If you are following the Eczema Detox Program, use the Eczema Detox food shopping list (p. 92–3) as a guide.

'I was told to eat fermented foods; why don't you recommend them in your book?'

Fermented foods are popular at the moment so try them if you like – just don't combine different treatments while following any of the programs in this book as it may affect your results.

Why I don't recommend fermented foods in this book is because adding histamine-rich fermented foods without first testing for histamine/amine intolerance is a risky 'one-size-fits-all' approach that can worsen eczema if you are histamine intolerant. More than 36 per cent of eczema sufferers adversely react to amines/histamines.[2] In this amine-sensitive group of people, eating fermented foods or probiotics will cause them to itch like crazy and flare up. *So test first, prescribe later.*

After completing the first three weeks of the FID Program, if you pass the amine test (p. 102) feel free to add fermented cabbage into your diet for three days to see how your skin responds (but avoid vinegar and other ingredients not permitted on this diet). After doing this test, if your skin worsens stop consuming fermented foods.

'Can I eat potatoes or will I react to them because they are nightshades?'

I don't know if you will adversely react to potatoes or any other food — the best way to find out is to test each food one by one (one new food every three days is the general rule). Only you can do this. Not everyone adversely reacts to nightshades and testing them is the best way to self-diagnose if a food is right for you. Read 'Additional tests' on p. 115 to find out how.

'What are the best types of potatoes to eat on the diet?'

If you are following the FID Program, only eat white potatoes, not cream/yellow or coloured. Most potatoes contain salicylates, especially the coloured ones. White potatoes (when thickly peeled) are low in salicylates but don't get them mixed up with the cream-coloured ones, which look off-white or slightly yellow when cut. White potatoes include Sebago, brushed (they are the ones usually sold with dirt on them), Kennebec and Coliban. Other white potatoes are available but you will need to cut them open to see if they are truly white. Low GI potatoes include Carisma, which may contain some salicylates (content is unknown). During the FID program avoid these potatoes: Baby, Desiree, Dutch cream, Golden, Kipfler, New, Nicola, Pontiac and all coloured potatoes, as they contain salicylates.[3]

Problem solving

'I have followed the Eczema Detox Program for the past two weeks and my skin is getting worse. Should I stop?'

It is a little too early to tell as it could be a detox reaction, which can occur for up to two weeks. If your skin does not start improving by three weeks, then switch to the FID Program so you can diagnose food intolerances and find out what is right for you.

'I have followed the Eczema Detox Program for two months and my skin has not improved. Should I stop?'

Yes, switch to the Food Intolerance Diagnosis Program (Chapter 8), as your skin should be improving by now. This is a sign you have undiagnosed food intolerances and the FID Program will help you identify them.

'I'm following the FID Program and I have done the tests, and I did not react to amines or salicylates but my skin is slowly getting worse. What do I do next?'

Investigate further. Are you sure you are not reacting to salicylates or amines? If your skin is worsening during testing it could be a sign you are sensitive to salicylates or amines or something else you are consuming. Note that reactions can be slow to appear, so diagnosis can be difficult. Keeping a diet diary can help (download one via www.eczemalife.com).

I suggest rotating your diet by trying the gluten-free FID menu on p. 100–1, to check for gluten intolerance. Refer to 'Additional tests' below to find out what to do next. Before you begin, here are some tips to help you make a clear diagnosis:

- Before each test, rate your eczema and itch out of 10. For example, 1–3 is good, 8–10 is bad etc.
- Take a photo of your eczema before you begin, so you have a reference to see if your skin improves or worsens during the testing phase.
- When doing the tests, eat two to three decent sized servings of the test food per day (ideally in the morning or with lunch in case you have a severe reaction). Using only small portions of a test food might make the results unclear.
- Then analyze the results: is your skin better or worse? Check your photos if you are unsure.
- Not all adverse reactions show up in the skin! Your skin might not have changed but check for other adverse reactions such as stomach issues, headaches, hyperactivity, fatigue, irritability, asthma, hay fever, a tight feeling in your throat etc. (Refer to the salicylate sensitivity symptoms in Chapter 1, p. 9.)
- If you experience an adverse reaction stop the testing and wait until your skin has calmed down before starting the next test. Avoid eating the 'problem' food for now and test it again in eight weeks' time, if desired.
- Avoid this test if you have anaphylactic reactions to anything or keep an EpiPen handy. If you have severe allergies, medical supervision may be required.

Additional tests

A guide to additional tests can be found in the table on the following pages. You can choose the order in which you test, and I suggest testing first the foods that you consume most often. You can stop the testing phase sooner if you have an adverse reaction.

Problem-solving: additional tests

Avoid for 5 days	Relevant program to follow	Test for 2–3 days (you might need to test for up to 7 days)
If you have been eating or drinking soy, avoid soy and soy lecithin and any supplements (such as vitamin D) that do not state they are 'soy free'.	Choose one of the FID menus (Chapter 10) and exclude soy. Do not test soy if you already know you adversely react to it.	Test soy for up to 3 days by eating 2–3 serves daily. Analyze the results.
Avoid gluten-containing foods including spelt, wheat, rye, oats, and check labels for gluten (or you can test one grain at a time, starting with spelt).	Follow the gluten-free FID menu for 5 days (see pp. 100–1).	Test gluten-rich spelt for 3 days (pancakes, spelt toast etc.). Are you better or worse? Check your photos if you are unsure. If your skin has not worsened then test oats for 3 days, then rye.
Avoid potatoes for 5 days (check all labels of packaged goods).	Choose one of the FID menus (Chapter 10) and exclude potatoes from your diet.	Test potatoes for 2–3 days. Analyze the results. If there is no adverse reaction, skip the starch test.
Avoid rice, rice malt syrup, rice bran oil etc.	Choose one of the FID menus (Chapter 10) and exclude rice from your diet. Substitute with quinoa or spelt if not sensitive to these.	Test rice for 2–3 days. Analyze the results. If there is no adverse reaction, skip the starch test.
Optional (depending on previous test results): avoid starch including potatoes, rice, oats, rye, spelt, barley, buckwheat, millet, quinoa.	Choose The Easy FID menu (pp. 96–7) and exclude starch from your diet. Increase protein and vegetable intake.	Test starch for 2–3 days. Analyze the results. You can test quinoa and buckwheat etc. separately to check for allergies.
Celery (allergy can occur in 1–9% of people with eczema).	Choose one of the FID menus (Chapter 10) and exclude celery from your diet.	Test celery for 3–7 days for accuracy. Analyze the results.
Avoid tannins, including pears, carob, vanilla and red cabbage.	Choose one of the FID menus (Chapter 10) and exclude tannin-rich foods from your diet.	Test tannins for 3–7 days. Analyze the results.
Fructose (anything sweet e.g. rice syrup, pear and maple syrup).	Choose one of the FID menus (Chapter 10) and exclude rice from diet.	Test fructose for 3–7 days. Analyze the results.

Avoid for 5 days	Relevant program to follow	Test for 2–3 days (you might need to test for up to 7 days)
Avoid meat (go vegan).	Choose Easy FID menu (p. 96–7), exclude meats from diet and have vegetarian/ vegan options.	Test cooked fresh meats (not deli meats) for 3 days. Analyze the results.
Avoid FODMAPs (this is usually a test for people with gut symptoms), including pear, Brussels sprouts, cabbage, garlic, leeks, legumes, shallots (spring onions/scallions), beans, legumes, garlic powder, choko (chayote), celery, soy and cashews.	If you are not sensitive to salicylates follow the Eczema Detox Program (Chapter 9) or the FID Program (Chapter 8) and exclude FODMAPs for up to 10 days.	Test FODMAPs for up to 7 days, especially leeks and other ingredients that you have not individually tested. Stop the test if you react. Check your photos if you are unsure.
Egg (cooked only).	You have already been avoiding egg on the program.	Test egg for 3 days. Analyze the results.
Once your eczema completely clears up you might want to test dairy. Do not test it too early as it could affect your results.	You have already been excluding dairy products from your diet.	Test high amounts of dairy for 3–7 days, especially milk and yoghurt. Analyze the results.

If you wish to test wheat, test it after you have completed the 12-week program or when your skin has cleared up. If you are still unsure how to conduct food intolerance tests, enlist the help of a nutritionist or dietician who specializes in food and chemical intolerances. Keep investigating until you find your trigger foods – you'll know you are on the right track when your skin clears up. If you need extra help you can contact my support team via support@eczemalife.com.

'I am allergic to gluten, dairy and egg and sensitive to salicylate, soy and amines; what can I eat and how do I reverse my intolerances so I can get more variety in my diet?'

Don't worry, there are plenty of suitable recipes in this book and there is a gluten-free FID menu on pp. 100–1 that you can follow, plus extra recipes you can adapt to make gluten-free. The Skin Supplement Program and the diet will help to reverse food intolerances, so be patient and hang in there as it may take time. If you need support along the way, join our Eczema Diet support group as our members share tips and recipes (see 'Useful resources', p. 220).

How to manage amine intolerance

'I have amine intolerance, so what foods should I avoid and do I have to avoid every single amine food?'

You will need to work out your own threshold — i.e. what types of amine foods you can tolerate. Some people are highly sensitive and need to strictly avoid every amine-containing food, while others can tolerate medium amine foods (refer to medium list) or small servings. However, while you have eczema begin by being strict.

Some other tips include:

» learn to cook (if you haven't already) so you can mostly eat freshly prepared foods, instead of leftovers
» take Skin Friend AM as it contains anti-histamine vitamins and will help you to recover from amine intolerance
» eat the recipes in this book, especially the ones in the FID Program, but avoid bananas, Therapeutic Broth, leftover cooked meats, frozen fish, salmon, papaya and pawpaw, as they contain amines.

Avoid foods rich/high in amines

Alcoholic drinks, anchovies, artificial food colourings, avocado, bacon, benzoate (preservative), bologna, broad beans (fava beans), broccoli, meat-based broth, buttermilk, cacao, canned tuna, cauliflower, cheese (all types), chicken skin/liver, chocolate (especially dark), cocoa powder, coconut, coconut oil, cola drinks, curry powder, dates, deli meats, eggplant (aubergine), extra virgin olive oil, fermented foods, figs, fish roe, frankfurters, fish that is frozen, salted, smoked or pickled, gherkin (pickles), grapes, gravy, green tea, ham, hydrolyzed vegetable protein, kefir, kiwi fruit, leftover meats, lemons, mandarin, matcha tea, meat extracts, miso, mushrooms, nuts (most, except raw cashews; avoid roasted cashews), offal, olive oil, olives, orange, orange juice, passionfruit, pepperoni, pickled foods, pineapple, plum, pork, probiotics, prunes, raisins/sultanas, red beans, reheated meat, salami, salmon, sardines, sauerkraut, sausages, sesame oil, smoked meats, soy sauce/ tamari sauce, spinach, stock cubes, strawberries, sugar/ladyfinger bananas, sulphites, most takeaway (takeout) meals, tartrazine (food colour), tea (black), tempeh, tomato, tomato sauces, tomato juice, tuna, vinegar (all types, but malt vinegar has lower), walnut oil, yeast extracts, yeasted products, yoghurt (all types).

Note: histamines have also been detected in raspberries, apricots, cherries, pumpkin (winter squash), shellfish and most types of fish except for fresh white fish.

Limit (or avoid) foods that have a medium level of amines

Banana, chia seeds, papaya, pawpaw and flaxseeds/linseeds (note flaxseed oil is an important source of omega-3 and contains fewer amines than the whole seed, and ¼ to ½ teaspoon daily is usually well tolerated by people with amine sensitivity).

Avoid histamine liberators

Additives/colourings, benzoates, cacao, citric fruits, chocolate, cocoa, glutamates (e.g. MSG), nitrites (e.g. ham), nuts, raw egg whites and sulphites (preservative, often sprayed on grapes and can be hidden in multivitamin supplements).

As mentioned, if you have been diagnosed with amine intolerance you need to work out your threshold of intolerance (i.e. the quantity of amine foods you can eat without adverse reaction). So begin by avoiding all amine foods, then one by one try ¼ to ½ teaspoon of flaxseed oil and other medium amine foods in very low amounts. Each month test new foods and note your skin's response. The goal is to gradually expand your diet and be eczema-free, so keep following this book as long as you need to.

How to manage and prevent salicylate intolerance

Some people are highly sensitive to salicylates and find their skin clears up when they strictly avoid salicylate-containing foods, while many others can tolerate moderate amounts in their diet. This book will help you work out your tolerance level. Some tips include:

»   Begin by using the FID Program recipes (from p. 124) and food shopping list (p. 78).
»   Take Skin Friend AM and PM as they contain the specific nutrients that enhance salicylate detoxification and tolerance.
»   Depending on your tolerance level, you may also need to avoid foods and beverages containing *moderate* (medium) amounts of salicylates — for a list of these foods refer to the Eczema Detox food shopping list on pp. 92–3.

Salicylate-rich foods and beverages

After your skin improves, gradually test salicylate-rich foods and expand your diet. In the meantime, if you are sensitive to salicylates, avoid the following foods and beverages

FRUITS (HIGH)

Apple, apricot, berries (all), rockmelon (cantaloupe), cherry, fig, guava, lemon, lime, lychee, nectarine, peach, pomegranate, strawberry, sugar/ladyfinger banana (regular bananas are okay), watermelon and other melons.

FRUITS (VERY HIGH!)

Avocado, cranberry, currant, date, dried fruit (all), grapefruit, grape, kiwi fruit, loganberry, mandarin, orange, passionfruit, pineapple, plum, raspberry, tangelo, tangerine and tomato.

VEGETABLES AND HERBS (HIGH)

Alfalfa sprouts, artichoke, basil, capsicum (bell pepper), chicory, chilli (chili pepper), corn, cucumber, endive (chicory, wiltof), herbs (most*), kale, okra, onion, pepper, radish, rocket (arugula), rosemary, spices (most*), thyme, turmeric, water chestnut, watercress and zucchini (courgette).

*If it's not on the shopping lists, it's high in salicylates.

VEGETABLES (VERY HIGH!)

Eggplant (aubergine), broad beans (fava beans), broccoli, cauliflower, mushroom, olive, pickled vegetables, silverbeet and spinach.

NUTS AND SEEDS (HIGH)

Almonds, Brazil nut, cashew nut (roasted, not raw), coconut, hazelnut, macadamia nut, peanut, pecan, pine nut, pistachio, pumpkin seed (pepitas), sesame seed, sunflower seed and walnut.

MEAT AND FISH (VERY HIGH!)

Devon, frankfurters/hotdogs, meat pies, processed lunch meats (chicken, turkey, etc.), salami, sausages, seasoned meats, tuna in olive oil or flavoured. (Enjoy fresh, unseasoned meats and most fresh white fish as they are salicylate-free.)

CONDIMENTS (VERY HIGH!)

Apple cider vinegar, bouillon (stock cubes), curry powder, gravies, honey, jam, jellies, most dips, sauces, tomato sauce, Vegemite and vinegar.

OTHER (HIGH TO VERY HIGH!)

Alcohol (except for gin, vodka and whiskey), beer, chewing gum, cider, cordials, fruit juices, green tea, herbal medicines, herbal teas, many supplements, peppermint, soft drinks/sodas (flavoured), Spirulina, tea, toothpaste (flavoured) and wheatgrass. (Decaffeinated coffee is low in salicylates and okay in moderation, but avoid coffee as it contains caffeine and moderate salicylates.)[4]

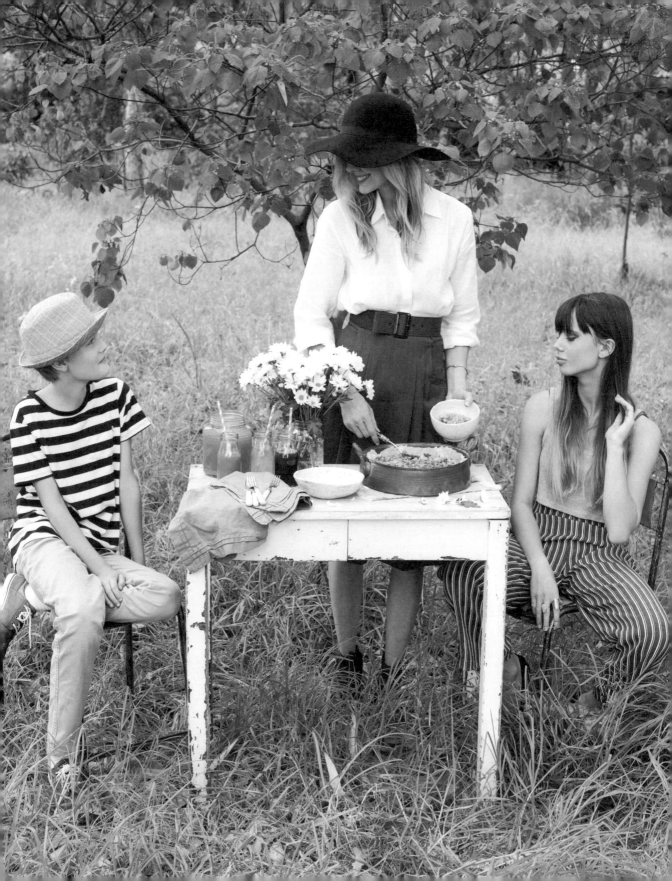

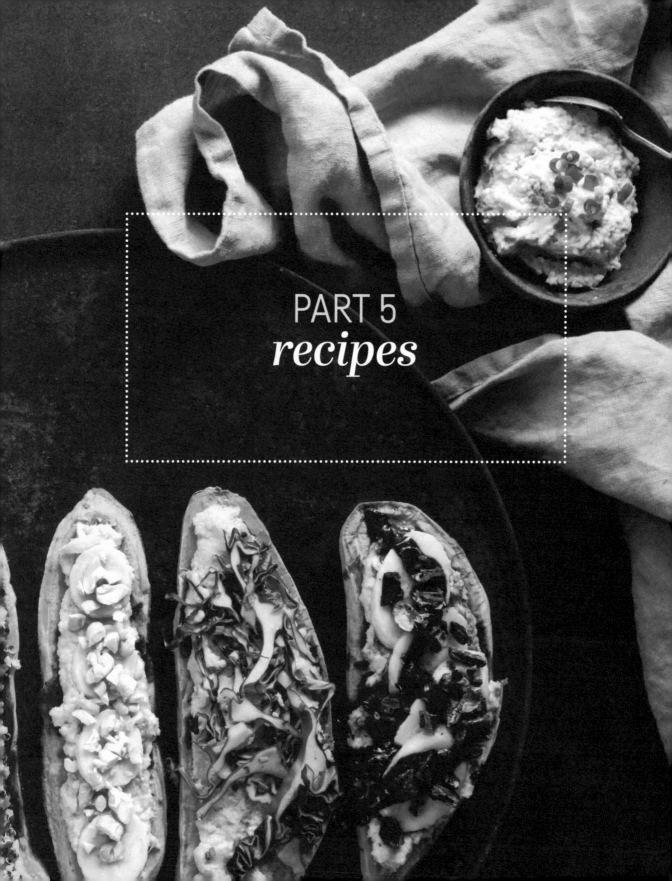

PART 5
recipes

Volume equivalents

Metric	Imperial (approximate)
20 ml	½ fl oz
60 ml	2 fl oz
80 ml	3 fl oz
125 ml	4½ fl oz
160 ml	5½ fl oz
180 ml	6 fl oz
250 ml (1 cup)	9 fl oz
375 ml	13 fl oz
500 ml	18 fl oz
750 ml	27 fl oz
1 L	25 fl oz

Weight equivalents

Metric	Imperial (approximate)
10 g	⅓ oz
50 g	2 oz
80 g	3 oz
100 g	3½ oz
150 g	5 oz
175 g	6 oz
200 g	7 oz
250 g	9 oz
375 g	13 oz
400 g	14 oz
500 g	1 lb
750 g	1 lb 10 oz
1 kg	2 lb

Oven temperatures

°Celsius (C)	°Fahrenheit (F)
120	235
150	300
180	350
200	400
220	425

Symbols			
detox	Eczema Detox Program recipe	s	contains moderate salicylates
fid	FID Program recipe	ss	contains high salicylates
veg	recipe is suitable for everyone, including vegans and vegetarians	aa	contains high amines
a	contains moderate amines	gf	recipe is gluten-free

The recipes in this book have been sorted into 'FID' for low-chemical recipes, 'Detox' which contain some foods with moderate levels of amines and salicylates, and 'Test', which is the test recipes for the FID Program. For all low-chemical recipes see the 'fid' dots above the recipes; for moderate-chemical recipes, see the 's' or 'a' dots; and for the high-chemical recipes see the 'ss' and 'aa' dots above the recipe.

This is a compilation of my favourite recipes. They contain a variety of healthy low-chemical and low-salicylate ingredients.

My daughter and I are no longer sensitive to salicylates but we still make the recipes from this book every week because we truly love them. Like us, I hope you enjoy the recipes and refer to them, like old friends, long after your eczema has cleared up.

Chapter 13
Recipes: FID Program

Drinks

It's incredibly important to hydrate throughout the day, especially if you have skin problems. These specially crafted recipes are naturally low in chemicals and rich in vitamins and minerals and other gentle, healthy ingredients to help you on your road to clear skin. These recipes are suitable for children and adults who are following the FID Program or Eczema Detox Program.

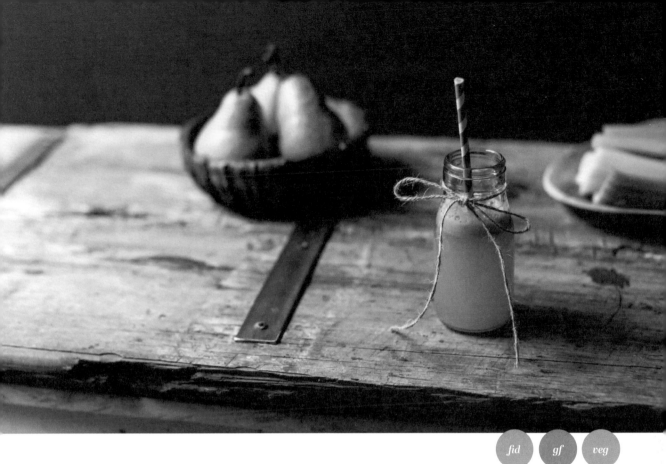

Celery Cleansing Juice

Serves 2, preparation time 5 minutes

For super-sensitive individuals, this drink is low in natural chemicals and is designed to restore the acid–alkaline balance in the body and aid liver detoxification. Adjust measurements to suit your tastes.

- 5 stalks celery
- ¼ head iceberg lettuce
- 1 large pear (must be ripe, not Nashi/Asian or Ya)
- 1 handful mung bean sprouts (freshest only, thoroughly washed)
- filtered water
- Skin Friend AM (optional)

Wash the vegetables and peel the pear. Using a juicing machine, juice the ingredients, ending by adding a splash of filtered water. Whisk in the vitamin powder if desired.

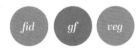

Carob Tea

Serves 1, preparation time 2 minutes

- 1 teaspoon carob powder
- 1 teaspoon (or to taste) rice malt syrup (brown rice syrup) or ½ teaspoon real maple syrup
- rice milk
- Skin Friend AM or PM (optional)

Pour boiling water into a tea or coffee cup, to fill about ¾ of the cup. Add the carob powder, rice malt syrup and top with rice milk, and mix well.

Optional: if making this tea in the morning, add Skin Friend AM or for an afternoon drink add Skin Friend PM. Check the drink is not too hot before adding Skin Friend AM as hot water will destroy the B vitamins and vitamin C.

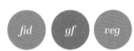

Pear and Vanilla Tea

Serves 6, preparation time 4 minutes, cooking time 10 minutes

Vanilla in tea is known to alleviate digestive problems, reduce tension in the body, and increase feelings of satiety and pleasure. This delicious sweet tea has a lovely aroma, and is made in bulk so you have a quick and easy supply on hand. This recipe makes great iced tea too.

- 8 cups filtered water
- 3 ripe pears (not Nashi, Asian or Ya), peeled, diced,
  core removed
- 1 vanilla bean
- 1 teaspoon rice malt syrup (brown rice syrup) or real maple syrup (optional)

In a large saucepan bring the water to the boil and add the pear. Cut a slit in the vanilla bean lengthways and add the vanilla bean to the brew and simmer for 10 minutes with the lid on. If you would like a sweet tea, stir in the rice malt syrup, to taste.

Using a slotted spoon remove the pears and store them in a sealed container for snacks. Store the leftover tea in a jug in the fridge.

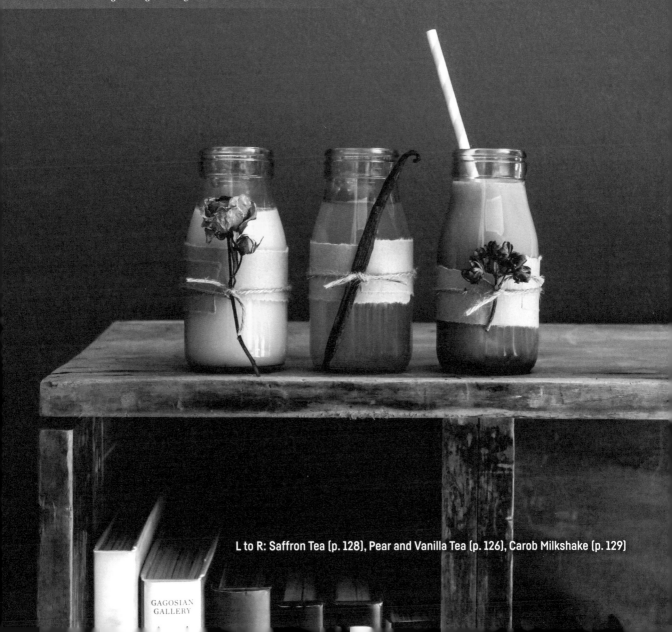

Carob is a great chocolate-free substitute. It improves digestion and helps you to feel satisfied as it inhibits the hormone ghrelin, which makes you feel hungry. It also tastes great. And it's rich in antioxidants, calcium, magnesium, vitamin B2, vitamin B6 and dietary fibre. It's also free of salicylates and amines.

L to R: Saffron Tea (p. 128), Pear and Vanilla Tea (p. 126), Carob Milkshake (p. 129)

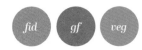

Saffron Tea

Serves 1, preparation time 1 minute, cooking time 5 minutes

Saffron is a natural antihistamine spice, which has been used for centuries as a digestive aid for people with gut issues.

- 1½ cups rice milk (or organic soy milk or oat milk)
- 5 threads (approx.) of saffron

Place the rice milk and saffron threads into a small saucepan and bring to the boil then reduce heat and simmer on low for 5 minutes to infuse. Pour into a mug and consume warm.

Notes:
- Saffron threads will not dissolve but can be eaten.
- Ideally, do not add sweetener as rice milk is sweet, but you can add a little real maple syrup or rice malt syrup (brown rice syrup) if needed.

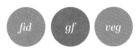

Electrolyte Pear Juice

Serves 4, preparation time 5 minutes, cooking time 5 minutes.

Hydrate your body with this natural electrolyte juice, which is ideal to use before or after exercise or for extra hydration once a day. Real maple syrup is rich in minerals including potassium, calcium, manganese and zinc. Potassium, sodium, calcium and magnesium are natural electrolytes.

- 6 cups filtered water
- 2 ripe pears, peeled, core removed and sliced (not Nashi/Asian or Ya pears)
- 1 pinch quality sea salt
- 1 teaspoon real maple syrup/brown rice syrup (or to taste)
- 1 g (1 scoop) fine calcium powder (optional, see 'Useful resources' on p. 220)

In a medium-sized saucepan, bring the water to the boil, then add the pear and salt and simmer for 5 minutes. Remove the saucepan from the heat, place the pear water and pears in a container and refrigerate until cool. Add the maple syrup and calcium powder then, using a high-powered blender, blend it in batches until smooth. Refrigerate and use as needed.

Carob Milkshake (hot or cold)

Serves 1 adult or 2 children, preparation time 2 minutes

This drink is suitable as a treat or bedtime drink for improving sleep. Carob is naturally sweeter than chocolate, it is caffeine-free and low in chemicals, making it ideal for eczema sufferers. Do not use cocoa or cacao as substitutes as they contain caffeine and can dry out your skin and hamper sleep.

- 1 teaspoon carob powder (add more if desired)
- 1 teaspoon rice malt syrup (brown rice syrup) or real maple syrup (optional, it may not need sweetening)
- 1½ cups organic gluten-free soy or rice milk (see 'Non-dairy milks', p. 52)
- 1 g (1 scoop) fine calcium powder (optional, to improve sleep)

Cold milkshake: The secret to a lump-free drink is to mix the carob powder and rice syrup in a tablespoon of boiling hot water before adding it to the milk. Alternatively, combine all the ingredients in a blender and blend on high until smooth.

Warm drink: Heat the milk in a small saucepan over medium heat. Meanwhile, mix the carob powder and rice syrup with a tablespoon of boiling water, then add it to the milk and stir until heated.

Notes:
- For calcium powder information refer to p. 183 and 'Useful resources' on p. 220.
- Optional: if making a cold milkshake, decorate the glass with Carob Syrup (p. 134) before pouring in the milkshake and top with extra carob syrup (pure carob syrup can also be bought online).

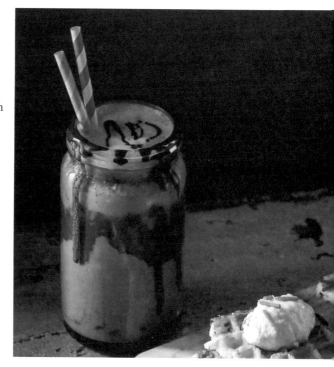

Dips, dressings, sauces and jams

These carefully crafted condiments for the FID Program are not only delicious, they are also low in chemicals and rich in a powerful combination of nutrients for healthy skin. If you are following the Eczema Detox Program you can also enjoy these condiments as they will make your program extra delicious.

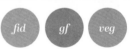

Caramelized Leek Sauce

Makes 4 servings, preparation time 5 minutes, cooking time 10 minutes

- 1 small leek, green part removed (about 2 cups chopped)
- 1 tablespoon Parsley Oil (p. 134)
- 2 tablespoons real maple syrup (adjust to taste)
- quality sea salt, to taste

Thoroughly wash the leek layers to ensure they are free of dirt. Finely chop the white parts and palest green parts of the leek. Heat the oil in a saucepan on medium heat and sauté the leek until very soft and slightly golden. Add the syrup and sea salt to taste and cook on low heat for another few minutes until sticky and golden. Leftovers will keep for five days in the refrigerator.

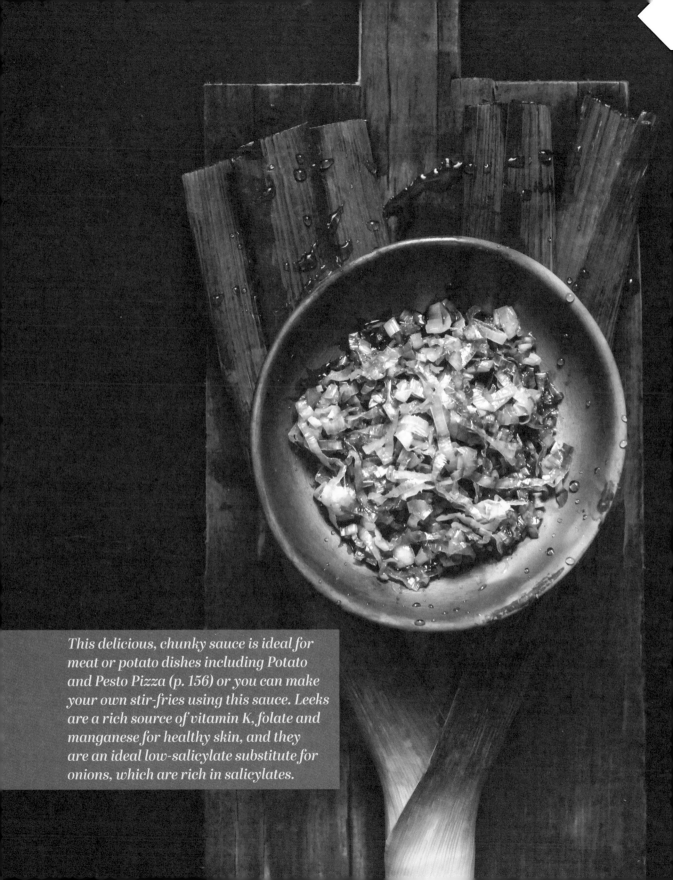

This delicious, chunky sauce is ideal for meat or potato dishes including Potato and Pesto Pizza (p. 156) or you can make your own stir-fries using this sauce. Leeks are a rich source of vitamin K, folate and manganese for healthy skin, and they are an ideal low-salicylate substitute for onions, which are rich in salicylates.

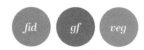

Bean Dip

Serves 6, preparation time 10 minutes
(if cooking beans fresh there is additional soaking and cooking time)

Kidney beans are a great source of fibre and the mineral molybdenum, which is responsible for detoxifying sulphites (see p. 14). Serve on toast or waffles, or with plain rice crackers or celery sticks.

- 1½ cups cooked kidney beans; see p. 171 for cooking instructions or use 1 x 400 g (14 oz) can red kidney beans or white beans such as navy (haricot) beans, drained and rinsed
- 1 small clove garlic, ½ teaspoon when minced
- 1 tablespoon Parsley Oil (p. 134)
- 4 tablespoons filtered water

Ensure you drain and rinse the beans before use. Place all the ingredients into a blender and blend, adding extra water if necessary to make a smooth paste. Store leftovers in a sealed container in the refrigerator for up to four days.

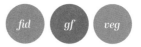

Sesame-free Hummus

Serves 6, preparation time 10 minutes
(if cooking chickpeas fresh there is additional soaking and cooking time)

- 1½ cups cooked chickpeas (garbanzo beans); see p. 171 for cooking instructions or use 1 x 400 g (14 oz) canned chickpeas, drained and rinsed
- 4–5 tablespoons filtered water
- 1 tablespoon Parsley Oil (p. 134)
- ¼ teaspoon garlic powder (optional)
- ½ teaspoon quality sea salt, or to taste

Note: add ½ clove garlic, minced (optional)

Place all the ingredients into a food processor and blend until smooth. Taste and adjust seasoning if necessary. Add a splash of water if a thinner consistency is desired. Hummus will last for four to five days in the refrigerator if stored in a sealed container.

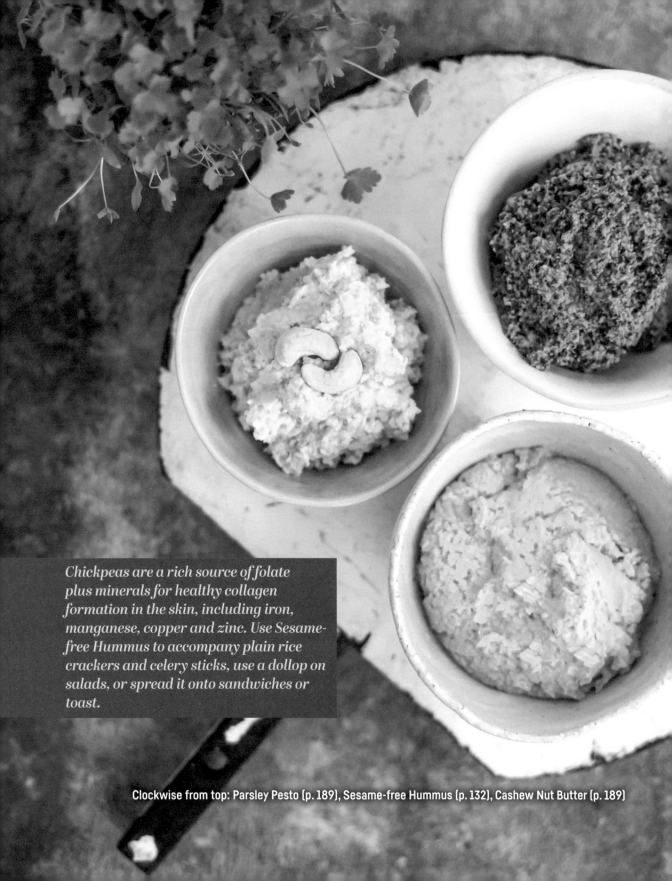

Chickpeas are a rich source of folate plus minerals for healthy collagen formation in the skin, including iron, manganese, copper and zinc. Use Sesame-free Hummus to accompany plain rice crackers and celery sticks, use a dollop on salads, or spread it onto sandwiches or toast.

Clockwise from top: Parsley Pesto (p. 189), Sesame-free Hummus (p. 132), Cashew Nut Butter (p. 189)

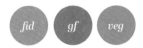

Carob Syrup

Makes 8+ servings, preparation time 5 minutes, cooking time 15 minutes

This lovely, thick caffeine-free sauce makes a decadent topping for desserts, or add it to warm rice milk for a calming bedtime drink. Carob is soothing to the digestive tract, it contains calcium to aid sleep, plus a tannin called gallic acid which has beneficial anti-allergic, antioxidant, antibacterial, antiseptic and antiviral properties. If you are sensitive to arrowroot flour, use fine rice flour.

- 1 cup filtered water
- ½ cup carob powder, sifted
- 2 teaspoons real maple syrup or rice malt syrup (brown rice syrup)
- 1 vanilla bean, cut lengthways and scraped (optional)
- 1 teaspoon arrowroot flour (to thicken)
- 1 tablespoon filtered water (additional)

Boil the filtered water in the kettle then add it to a small saucepan along with the carob powder, maple syrup and vanilla bean (if using), and simmer for about 10 minutes on low heat.

In a small cup, mix the arrowroot flour and tablespoon of water until it is lump-free. Then add this to the carob syrup and mix over a low heat until the syrup thickens. Remove from the heat and store in a sealed jar in the refrigerator.

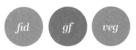

Parsley Oil

Makes ½ jar, preparation time 4 minutes

Parsley contains protective antioxidants that help to reduce the formation of glycation end-products, which can form when meats are cooked. Use this oil to baste chicken or lamb before roasting or grilling (broiling), or use it any time a recipe requires cooking oil.

- 2 teaspoons fresh parsley
- ½ cup rice bran oil (see notes)

Blanch the parsley in hot water for about 1 minute, then drain and dry with paper towels. Combine the parsley and oil in a high-powered blender until well blended. Then strain the oil using cheesecloth or muslin. Store in an airtight jar in the refrigerator and use within a couple of weeks.

Notes:

- If you are sensitive or allergic to rice or rice bran oil, use other low-salicylate oils such as sunflower oil or refined safflower oil.
- Important: check the oil does not contain artificial antioxidants such as E310–312, E319, E320 (BHA) and E321 (BHT) — they will make you itch like crazy.

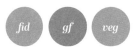

Maple Dressing

Makes 4 servings, preparation time 5 minutes

This sweet dressing is rich in minerals including potassium, calcium, manganese and zinc. It looks like balsamic dressing but without the acidic vinegar. It has the goodness of carob powder and immune-system balancing garlic. Try it on salads including the Wombok Noodle Salad on p. 175.

- ⅓ cup filtered water
- ¼ cup real maple syrup
- 4 teaspoons raw carob powder
- 4 teaspoons Parsley Oil (p. 134)
- ½ teaspoon quality sea salt (or less)
- 1 small clove garlic (optional)

Place the ingredients into a sealable jar and shake well to combine or place them into a blender. Stir or shake well before serving. Store the leftovers in the refrigerator for up to a week.

Notes:
- Optional: add 1 tablespoon freshly chopped chives.
- You can use rice malt syrup (brown rice syrup) instead of maple syrup (note it is less sweet).
- If you have completed the FID Program and are not highly sensitive to salicylates or sulphites, you can add 1 tablespoon malt vinegar to this recipe for extra tang and for preserving. If you want to test malt vinegar, consume it for up to three days to see if your skin adversely reacts within one to three days.

How to sterilize jars

When making jams and sauces, store them in hot sterilized jars to prevent them from spoiling. Dirty jars or jars that have not been sterilized correctly allow mould to form in the jam and you'll need to throw the batch away if this occurs.

Sterilizing jars is easy. Here's how:

- Preheat the oven to 120°C (250°F).
- Wash jars and lids in soapy water (do not use plastic lids), rinse and place them on a baking tray, with lids facing up, and ensure the jars are not touching each other.
- Place in the oven for about 20 minutes.
- Using thick mittens, remove and immediately pour in the hot, freshly cooked jam or sauce (tip: food must be hot when placed into the hot jars), and then seal tightly with the lids.

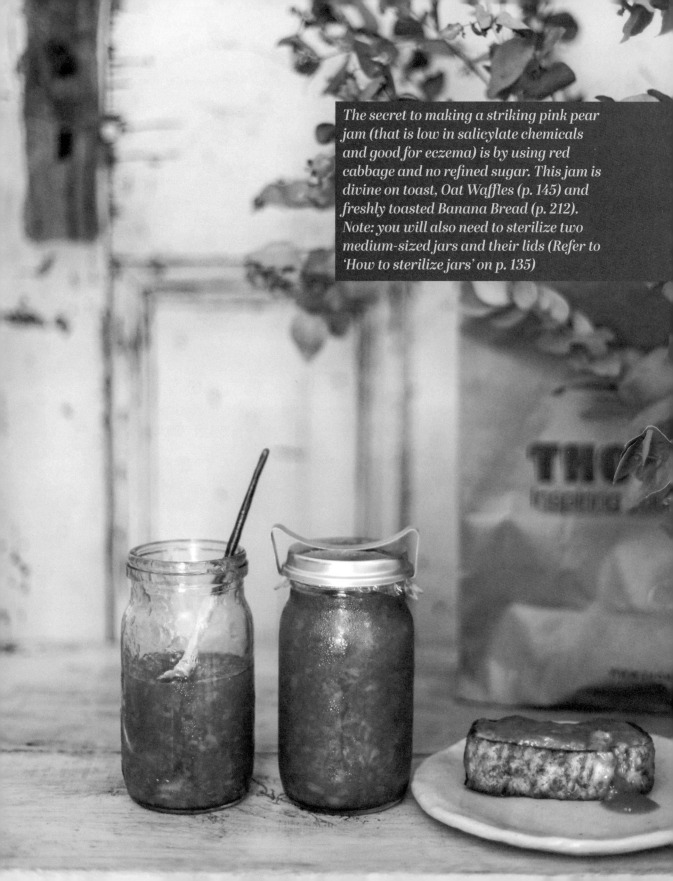

The secret to making a striking pink pear jam (that is low in salicylate chemicals and good for eczema) is by using red cabbage and no refined sugar. This jam is divine on toast, Oat Waffles (p. 145) and freshly toasted Banana Bread (p. 212). Note: you will also need to sterilize two medium-sized jars and their lids (Refer to 'How to sterilize jars' on p. 135)

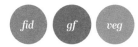

Pink Pear Jam

Makes 2 medium jars, preparation time 20 minutes, cooking time 30 minutes

- 12 ripe medium-sized pears (do not use Nashi/Asian or Ya)
- ¼ cup finely sliced purple/red cabbage
- ¼ cup filtered water
- ¾ cup rice malt syrup (brown rice syrup; see notes for alternatives)
- 1 or 2 x 50 g (2 oz) packet jam-setting agent (pectin) e.g. Jamsetta (one is a spare packet)

Place a small freezer-safe dish into the freezer.

Peel and dice the pears (discard the cores) and place the fruit into a large saucepan with the red cabbage, filtered water and rice malt syrup. Cook on medium heat for 20 minutes or until very soft and the mixture has turned pink, stirring often and checking it doesn't burn (turn to low as needed). If the pears are ripe, they will soften easily. Then mash with a potato masher, add the jam-setting agent (pectin) and mix well. Cook for another 10 minutes on low to medium heat.

Meanwhile, place your jars into the oven to sterilize them or boil them in a large saucepan of water (refer to instructions, on p. 135). Then test if the jam will set: take the dish out of the freezer and place a teaspoon of jam onto it. If the jam is ready, it will soon thicken and crinkle when moved. If it's too thin and not setting, add another ½ packet (25 g/0.8 oz) of jam-setting agent to the saucepan of jam and cook it for an extra 5 minutes, stirring often.

Remove the jars from the oven and scoop the jam into the hot sterilized jars using clean utensils (jars must be hot). Seal with lids and allow to cool.

Notes:
- If you cannot find rice malt syrup (brown rice syrup) you can use ½ cup real maple syrup instead. Another alternative is barley syrup (note: barley contains gluten).
- Under-ripe pears contain salicylates so ensure the pears are ripe.
- If fresh, ripe pears are unavailable try using canned pears in sugar syrup (don't use canned pears 'in juice' as the juice contains salicylates). Drain the syrup and adjust the recipe if needed.
- As this jam is free of refined sugars, it will not preserve for as long as usual. So store both jars in the refrigerator and use within a few weeks once the jar is opened.
- If you are allergic or sensitive to cabbage, use grated beetroot (beets) to colour the jam (if you are not sensitive to salicylates).

Breakfast

When it's time to 'break the fast' choose something healthy, delicious and extra nutritious. These FID Program recipes are designed to suit all preferences, from high protein (low carb) to high fibre, sweet and delicious. You can also enjoy them as snacks or lunch if you prefer. I recommend favouring the oil-free recipes which are the porridge options and the steamed version of Protein Vegie Bowl.

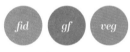

Beans on Toast

Serves 1–2, preparation time 10 minutes, cooking time 10 minutes
(extra time if you are making Alkaline Vegetable Broth)

- Optional: 2 slices spelt sourdough bread (buy wheat-free)
- ¼ cup filtered water or Alkaline Vegetable Broth (p. 167)
- ¼ leek, white part, finely chopped
- 1½ cups white beans (cannellini or navy/haricot)
- ¼ teaspoon quality sea salt or to taste
- ½ teaspoon garlic powder (optional)
- 1 tablespoon finely chopped chives (optional)

First, toast the bread if using. Meanwhile, heat the water or broth in a frying pan over medium heat. Add the leek and sauté until soft. Add the beans and mix with the leeks, smashing them a little with a wooden spoon. Continue cooking until the mixture thickens. Add salt, garlic powder and chives. Then remove from the heat and spoon the bean mixture onto toast.
Recipe by Charlie Rioux.

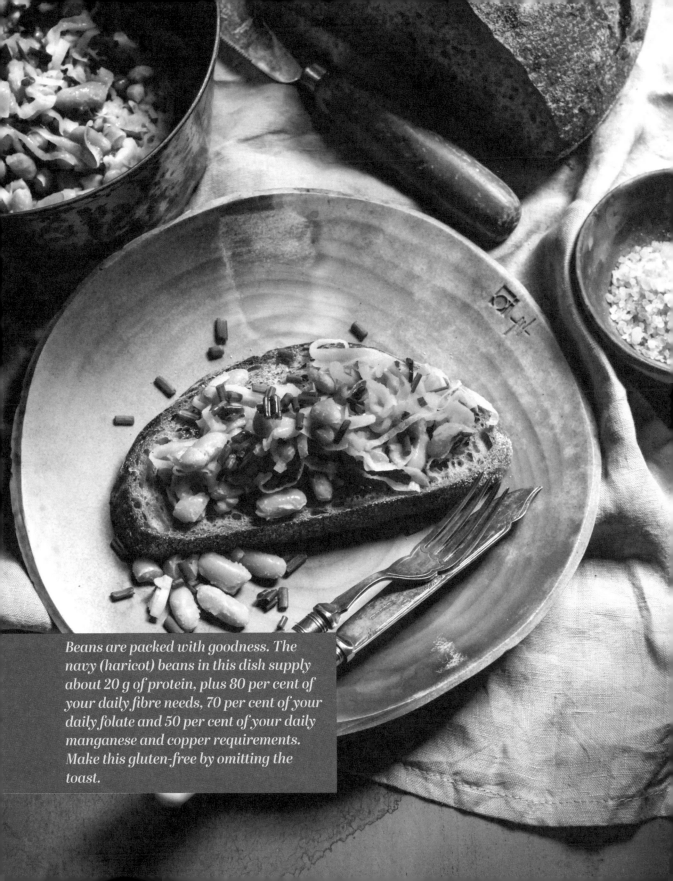

Beans are packed with goodness. The navy (haricot) beans in this dish supply about 20 g of protein, plus 80 per cent of your daily fibre needs, 70 per cent of your daily folate and 50 per cent of your daily manganese and copper requirements. Make this gluten-free by omitting the toast.

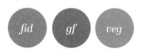

Protein Vegie Bowl

Serves 1, preparation time 10 minutes, cooking time 5 minutes

The vegetables can either be lightly steamed or briefly fried in a pan for a healthy, grain-free breakfast which is acid–alkaline balanced. I recommend using the steaming method to avoid using oil.

- ½ cup plain tofu, chopped (or free-range/ organic chicken if you prefer meat)
- sprinkle of quality sea salt
- sprinkle of garlic powder
- dried or fresh chives
- 1 teaspoon Parsley Oil (optional, p. 134)
- 1 small white potato, peeled and finely sliced
- ½ cup chopped red cabbage
- ½ cup green beans, ends trimmed and halved

Chop the tofu (or other protein option) into bite-sized pieces and coat them in a little salt, garlic powder and chives. Add the Parsley Oil to a small frying pan on medium heat and cook the protein until brown on each side (up to 2 minutes on each side — if cooking chicken, ensure it is well cooked through). Remove from the heat and drain on paper towels.

You have two options for cooking the vegetables. Steaming method: add 3 cm (1½ in) of boiling water to a saucepan, and place on top the steaming basket with the vegetables and cover with a lid. (Tip: separate the cabbage from the other vegetables as the purple will stain them.) Steam the vegetables for 2 minutes or until you can pierce the thickest piece with a fork, then remove from the heat. Do not overcook. Leave the cabbage and beans with a bit of crunch as they will continue to cook after removed from the heat.

If you wish to stir-fry the vegetables (instead of steaming), clean the frying pan and add a teaspoon of Parsley Oil. On medium to high heat, cook the sliced potato until it appears golden, flip the pieces over and repeat the process. Then lightly fry the cabbage and beans for 1 minute. Before serving, top the vegetables with chives and salt.

Spelt Pancakes

Makes 6–8 pancakes, preparation time 5 minutes, cooking time 15 minutes

Spelt is a nutritious ancient grain that is easier to digest than wheat. It's rich in dietary fibre, manganese, magnesium, zinc, selenium and B vitamins. Avoid spelt if you are allergic to gluten. This recipe is not suitable for days 1–14 of the FID Program (see notes).

- 1 cup spelt flour
- ¼ teaspoon bicarbonate of soda (baking soda)
- 1¼ cups organic soy milk or rice milk
- 1 egg (or use ½ ripe banana, peeled or make Egg Replacer — see notes)
- rice bran oil (or refer to 'Eczema-friendly cooking oils' on p. 50) for frying
- rice malt syrup (brown rice syrup) or real maple syrup
- 1–2 pears (avoid Asian/Nashi or Ya pears), peeled, (to serve) (if you are doing the Detox program, see notes)

Sift the flour and bicarbonate of soda into a mixing bowl and mix together. Gradually mix in the milk and stir until lump-free, then stir in the egg (or Egg Replacer, p. 211, or ½ banana, pureed). Heat a small non-stick frying pan, add a little oil, and using a ⅓ measuring cup pour the mixture into the pan. Lightly cook each side. Repeat until mixture is finished.

To serve, spread a thin layer of rice malt syrup or maple syrup onto the pancakes and top with pear.

Notes:
- If you have tested egg during the FID Program and there were no adverse reactions to eggs (within four days of testing), then you can use real egg in this recipe, or use ripe banana if you are not sensitive to amines, or make Egg Replacer (p. 211).
- If you are following the Eczema Detox Program (and if you are not sensitive to amines), you can top the pancakes with ripe papaya/pawpaw, banana, Banana Nice Cream (p. 216) or Papaya Nice Cream (p. 216).

Wholegrain Oat Porridge

Serves 1 adult, preparation time 5 minutes, cooking time 15 minutes

- ½ cup rolled oats (see notes for individual measurements)
- approx. 1½ cups filtered water
- ½ pear, peeled and thinly sliced (refer to photo) (avoid Asian/Nashi or Ya pears)
- 2–3 teaspoons real maple syrup or rice malt syrup (brown rice syrup)
- rice milk or non-dairy milk of choice from the list on p. 52, to serve

Rinse the oats with water and place them into a saucepan with the filtered water (aim for 1 part oats to 3 parts water). Bring to the boil and simmer on low heat for 10–15 minutes, stirring occasionally. Add extra water if necessary.

Meanwhile, lightly coat the pear slices in syrup. Heat a non-stick frying pan on medium heat and lightly fry the pears (no oil if possible), for about 2 minutes on each side, or until golden. Pour the cooked oats into a bowl and top with the pear and milk. If you would like sweetener, add rice malt syrup (brown rice syrup) or real maple syrup or Carob Syrup (p. 134).

Notes:

- Uncooked oat measurements: for adults, use ½ cup rolled oats each, older children use ⅓ cup each and for small children use ¼ cup each.
- Instant oats have a high glycaemic index (GI) which can lead to energy crashes later in the day, so favour rolled oats (also known as wholemeal oats) as these low GI varieties keep your blood sugar levels steady.
- If you are sensitive to oats, try the following recipe for Quinoa Porridge (p. 144).

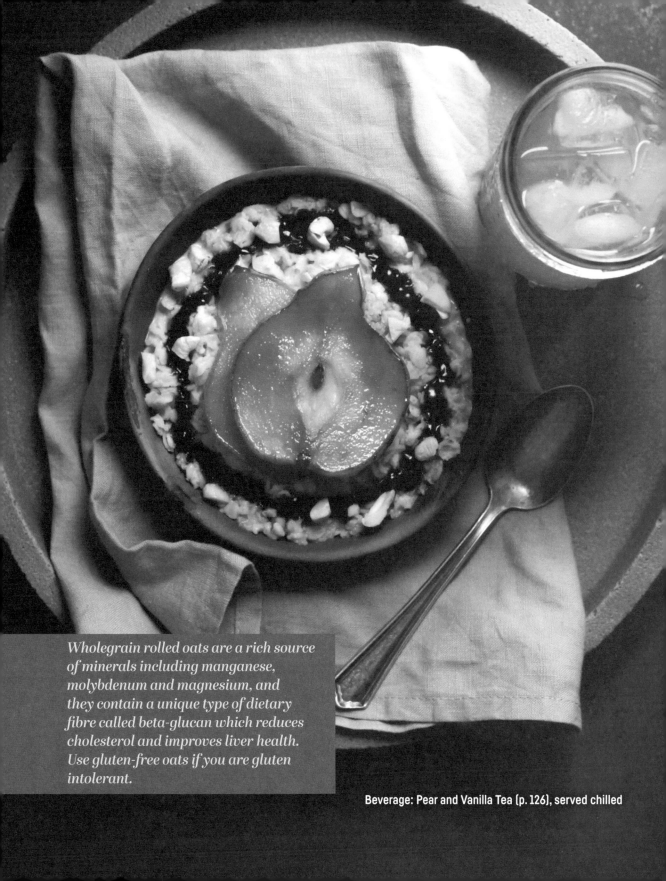

Wholegrain rolled oats are a rich source of minerals including manganese, molybdenum and magnesium, and they contain a unique type of dietary fibre called beta-glucan which reduces cholesterol and improves liver health. Use gluten-free oats if you are gluten intolerant.

Beverage: Pear and Vanilla Tea (p. 126), served chilled

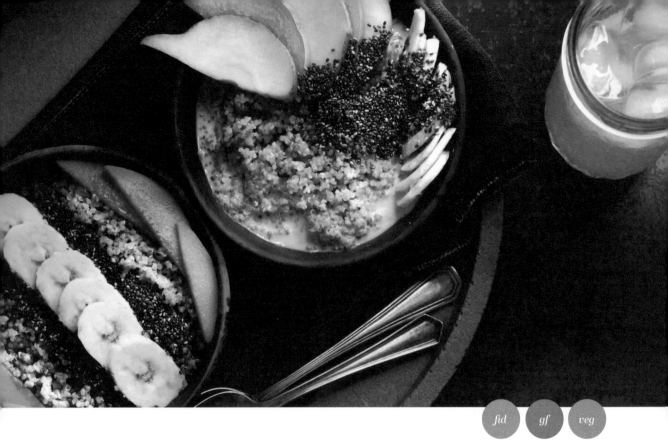

fid   gf   veg

Quinoa Porridge

Serves 1, preparation time 5 minutes, cooking time 20 minutes

Quinoa (pronounced 'keen-wah') is a gluten-free grain-like seed that contains more antioxidants than any other grain. Half a cup of quinoa provides about 78 mg magnesium, 5 g protein, 1.4 mg zinc and small amounts of omega-3 for healthy skin.

- ½ cup white quinoa, rinsed (do not use puffed quinoa)
- 1 cup filtered water
- ½ teaspoon real vanilla essence (optional)
- ½ cup organic malt-free soy milk or rice milk (see 'Non-dairy Milks', p. 52)
- pear, peeled, to serve (avoid Asian/Nashi or Ya pears)
- 1 teaspoon rice malt syrup (brown rice syrup) or real maple syrup

Rinse the quinoa with water, then place it into a saucepan with the water and bring to the boil. Cook over low heat until the porridge is thick and the grains are tender, about 12–15 minutes. Add the vanilla and milk and cook for another 5 minutes. Stir occasionally to prevent burning and add more milk or water if necessary. Serve with pear and syrup of choice.

Note: if you are following the Eczema Detox Program you can enjoy other toppings such as banana and papaya, as pictured.

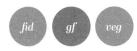

Oat Waffles

Serves 2, preparation time 5 minutes, cooking time 15 minutes

Oat waffles are a delicious and healthy bread substitute. Wholegrain rolled oats are a rich source of minerals and beta-glucan, which promotes liver health. Use gluten-free oats if you are gluten intolerant and add fresh alkalizing chives or parsley so the meal is acid–alkaline balanced.

- 1 cup rolled (wholegrain) oats
- 1 cup rice milk or oat milk
- 2 teaspoons Parsley Oil (p. 134)
- ½ teaspoon baking powder (gluten-free)
- 1 tablespoon finely chopped parsley (or dried)

Preheat the waffle iron on high heat. For crispy waffles, wait for the waffle iron to reheat in between batches.

Place the oats, rice milk, oil and baking powder into a blender and blend until smooth. Stir in the herbs. When the waffle iron is hot, ladle or pour the batter into the waffle maker, enough to cover the grid. Cook the waffles in batches until they are crisp and golden (about 5–7 minutes each). Serve immediately for crisp waffles as they tend to soften over time.

Notes:

- Ideally serve these waffles with fresh parsley and vegetables for acid-alkaline balance. Other options: serve with real maple syrup or Pink Pear Jam (p. 137) for sweet waffles. For savoury waffles serve with Sesame-free Hummus (p. 132) or Cashew Nut Butter (p. 189).
- Variation: add a tablespoon of carob powder for chocolaty waffles.
- Protein powder: if you are vegan or vegetarian (or want to increase your protein intake), add 1–2 tablespoons of pure pea/rice protein to the batter plus an extra ¼ cup milk. Do not use protein powder if you are sensitive to glutamates.

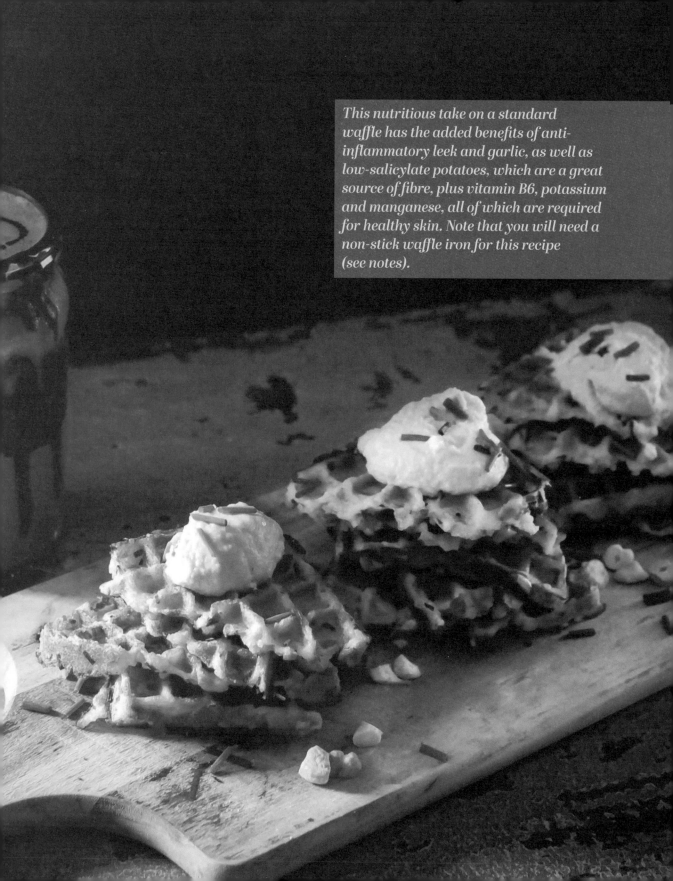

This nutritious take on a standard waffle has the added benefits of anti-inflammatory leek and garlic, as well as low-salicylate potatoes, which are a great source of fibre, plus vitamin B6, potassium and manganese, all of which are required for healthy skin. Note that you will need a non-stick waffle iron for this recipe (see notes).

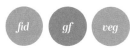

Potato and Leek Waffles

Makes 2 servings, preparation time 15 minutes, cooking time 30 minutes

- 2 heaped cups peeled and diced white potatoes, (2.5 cm/1-in cubes)
- 1 leek, white/light green parts only
- 1 clove garlic
- 3 teaspoons Parsley Oil (p. 134)
- ½ teaspoon sea salt
- ¼ cup brown rice flour (or flour to suit your allergies)
- 1 tablespoon chopped fresh chives (optional)

Steam or boil the potatoes until soft. Meanwhile, thoroughly wash the leek to remove any dirt from the layers and finely dice. Chop or mince the garlic clove.

Add 1–2 tablespoons of water to a frying pan over medium heat. Add the leek and garlic and sauté until soft. Set aside.

When the potatoes are cooked, drain and mash them using the same pot. Add the oil, salt and flour and mash until well combined.

Preheat the waffle iron (coat with oil if it is not completely non-stick; *ideally do not add more oil*, preferably use a new appliance to avoid sticking). Divide the potato mixture into two and form into discs. When the waffle iron is ready, add one disc to the centre of the iron, then slowly press down until the iron is closed. Cook until firm and crisp (about 5–7 minutes). Wait for the waffle iron to reheat then repeat.

Garnish with chopped chives and serve immediately for crisp waffles as they tend to soften over time.
Recipe by Charlie Rioux.

Note: if you are sensitive to salicylates be careful what sort of potatoes you buy. They must be the pure white varieties and thickly peeled (white potatoes are often called 'brushed potatoes' and they are usually sold with dirt on them). For more low-salicylate potatoes see the FID food shopping list on p. 78.

Snacks and lunchbox

The following FID Program recipes can be used as lunchbox items or for snacks between meals. If you are following the Eczema Detox Program you can also enjoy these recipes.

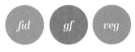

The Wishing Plate

Serves 2 as a light snack, preparation time 5 minutes

Choose from the following:

- 1 stalk celery, strings peeled, sliced into 'shark's teeth'
- mung bean sprouts (remove green shells if desired)
- cooked green beans (boiled for 1 minute)
- cooked red cabbage
- iceberg lettuce
- 1 carrot, peeled and chopped into sticks and circles (Eczema Detox Program; see notes)

Buy a decorative plate that you exclusively use as the Wishing Plate (e.g. a fairy plate or one suitable for the child's age and tastes). Each time your child eats two (or more) vegetables from the Wishing Plate they can make a wish. I encourage the whole family to join in. Leave this plate (covered) on the kitchen bench for everyone to use. Make it more convenient than junk food, serve it with the dips from this book, whatever you need to do to create positive eating habits.

Young children may want their vegies arranged into shapes (clock, truck, flower and so on) or they can create their own 'picture' arrangement before eating.

Note: as carrots contain moderate salicylates, exclude them during the first three weeks of the FID Program.

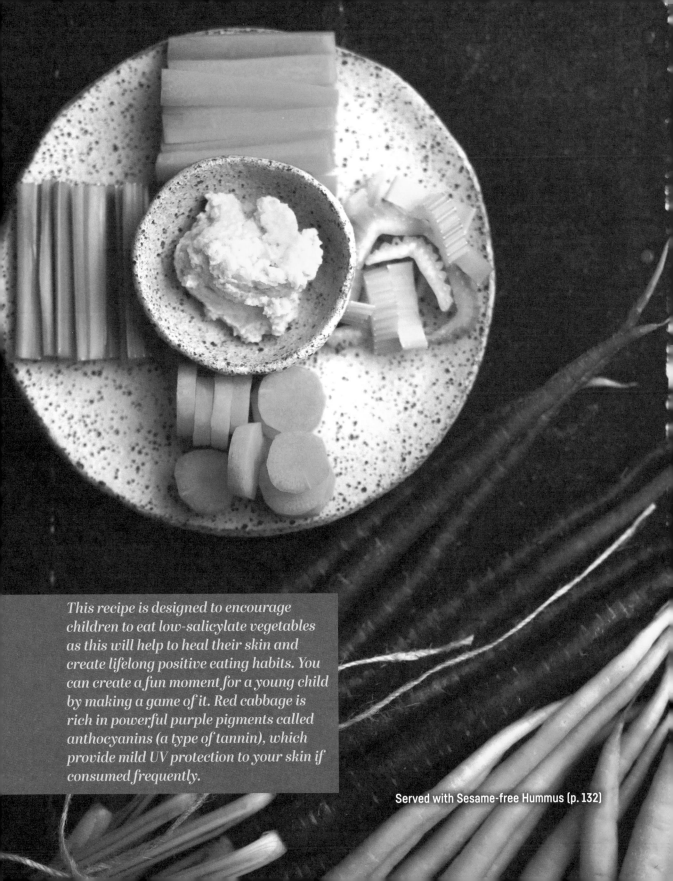

This recipe is designed to encourage children to eat low-salicylate vegetables as this will help to heal their skin and create lifelong positive eating habits. You can create a fun moment for a young child by making a game of it. Red cabbage is rich in powerful purple pigments called anthocyanins (a type of tannin), which provide mild UV protection to your skin if consumed frequently.

Served with Sesame-free Hummus (p. 132)

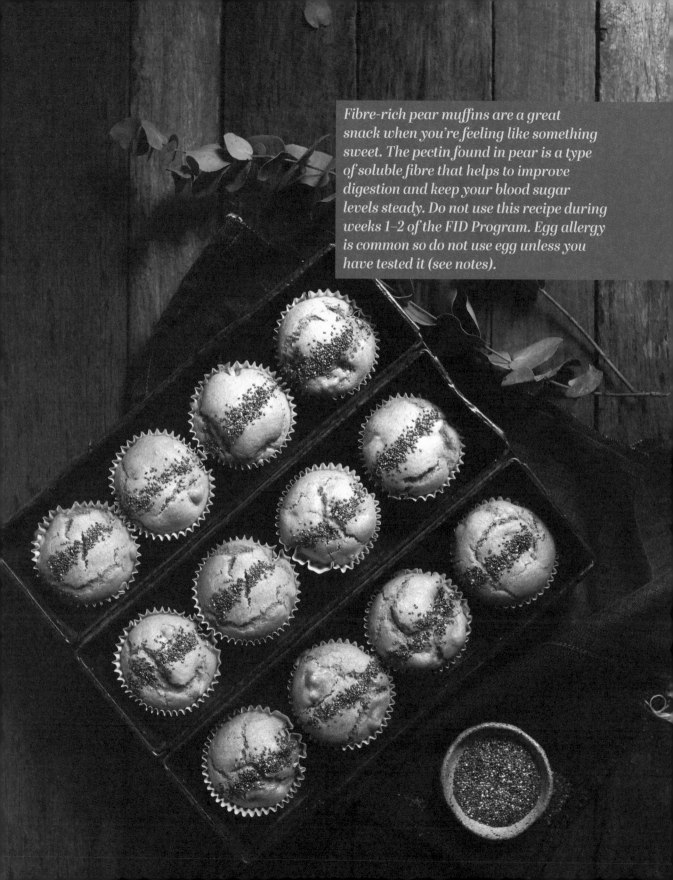

Fibre-rich pear muffins are a great snack when you're feeling like something sweet. The pectin found in pear is a type of soluble fibre that helps to improve digestion and keep your blood sugar levels steady. Do not use this recipe during weeks 1–2 of the FID Program. Egg allergy is common so do not use egg unless you have tested it (see notes).

Pear Spelt Muffins

Makes 12 muffins, preparation time 15 minutes, cooking time 15 minutes

- 1 egg (or use Egg Replacer, p. 211)
- ⅓ cup real maple syrup or maple sugar (see 'Eczema-friendly sweeteners', p. 52)
- 1 cup organic soy milk (see 'Non-dairy milks', p. 54)
- ⅓ cup Parsley Oil (p. 134) or rice bran oil
- 2 cups spelt flour
- 4 teaspoons baking powder (wheat-free)
- 2 large ripe pears, peeled and diced (not Nashi/Asian or Ya pears)

Preheat the oven to 180°C (350°F). Place paper patty pans into the holes of a 12-cup muffin tray (or alternatively grease the tray holes with a little extra rice bran oil).

If using Egg Replacer make it now. In a small food processor, blend the egg (or equivalent), maple syrup and milk until smooth. Then, while the motor is running, open the chute and slowly drizzle in the oil and blend well until smooth and creamy.

In a separate bowl, sift together the flour and baking powder and mix. Add the wet ingredients to the bowl with the dry ingredients and briefly mix using a large spoon. Then stir in the pear.

Spoon the mixture into each muffin cup, ensuring each is about three-quarters full. Bake for 15 minutes or until slightly golden on top. Test with a toothpick to see if cooked through.

Notes:
- These muffins can be stored in the freezer for up to three months.
- If you have tested egg during the FID Program (in week 3) and there were no adverse reactions after four days then you can use real egg in this recipe.
- If you are gluten intolerant, use rice milk or 'malt-free' soy milk and gluten-free self-raising flour instead of spelt flour. If you are using gluten-free self-raising flour, don't add baking powder.
- If you are following the Eczema Detox Program, you can sprinkle the muffins with chia seeds (see photo).

Spelt Chips

Serves 2–3, preparation time 5 minutes, cooking time 15 minutes

This simple recipe uses the delicious Spelt Flat Bread to make a great savoury snack or lunchbox item. Serve spelt chips with Sesame-free Hummus (p. 132) or Bean Dip (p. 132) if desired.

- Spelt Flat Bread (p. 155)
- quality sea salt, to taste

Preheat the oven to 180°C (350°F) and line a large shallow baking tray with baking paper.

Using two to three flat breads, cut each sheet in half then into 'corn chip' sized triangles. Sprinkle with a little salt and place the triangles onto the baking tray. Bake for 10–15 minutes or until hard and crispy. Store them in a sealed container in the cupboard for up to a week.

Lunch and dinner

An important part of healing your skin includes eating frequent meals — this includes eating lunch and dinner. Skipping these meals or having them late can cause unhealthy dips in your blood sugar levels, which can cause fatigue, anxiety and unhealthy cravings for sugar. A healthy body and mind needs frequent meals to function optimally. The following nutritious recipes are free from itch-promoting chemicals and have been designed to keep your blood sugar levels steady.

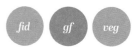

Alkaline Bomb Salad

Serves 1, preparation time 10 minutes

This is a strongly alkalizing vegetarian side salad and detox cleansing recipe. Mung bean sprouts are like little 'bombs' that help to alkalize the body. Ensure they are fresh and not going brown. It's incredibly easy to sprout your own (see p. 169 for instructions).

- 2 handfuls iceberg lettuce, shredded (or amount to suit you)
- 1 medium stalk of celery
- 1 spring onion (shallot, scallion), thinly sliced on the diagonal
- ¼ cup finely shredded red cabbage
- ¼ cup mung bean sprouts, rinsed and drained
- Sesame-free Hummus (p. 132) or Maple Dressing (p. 135)

Place the lettuce into a shallow bowl and top with the remaining ingredients, finishing with a large dollop of Sesame-free Hummus or a drizzle of dressing.

Notes:
- This salad can also be served with Spelt Flat Bread (p. 155).
- If you have thyroid problems, omit the cabbage.

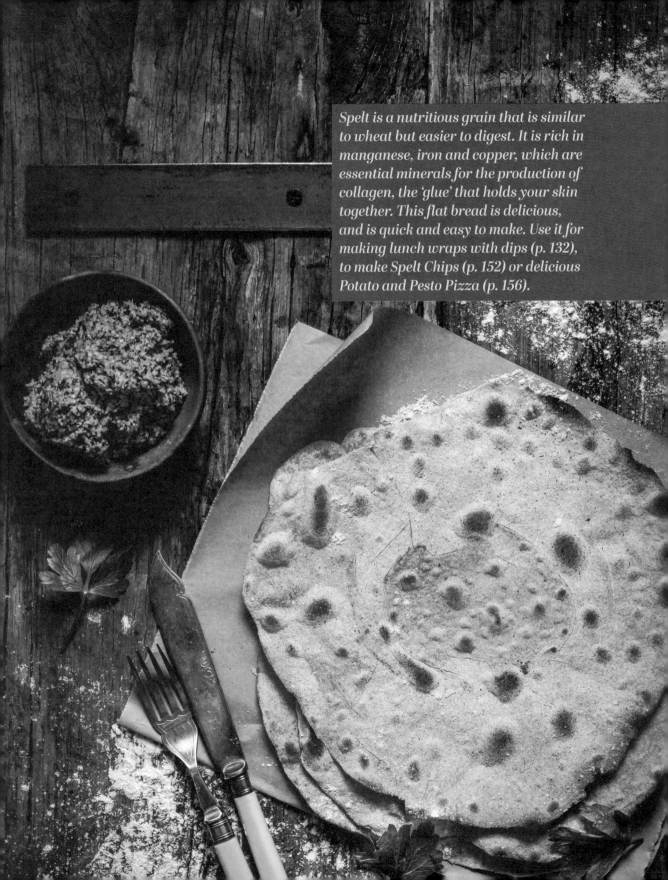

Spelt is a nutritious grain that is similar to wheat but easier to digest. It is rich in manganese, iron and copper, which are essential minerals for the production of collagen, the 'glue' that holds your skin together. This flat bread is delicious, and is quick and easy to make. Use it for making lunch wraps with dips (p. 132), to make Spelt Chips (p. 152) or delicious Potato and Pesto Pizza (p. 156).

Spelt Flat Bread

Makes 6, preparation time 10 minutes, cooking time 20 minutes

- 1¼ cups plain spelt flour, plus extra for kneading (wholemeal if available)
- ¾ teaspoon finely ground quality sea salt
- 1 tablespoon Parsley Oil (p. 134)
- ⅔ cup boiling water

In a bowl, mix together the spelt flour and salt. Add the oil and hot water, and mix using a knife. The dough should not be sticky — if it is, add extra flour until it can be kneaded without sticking to the board.

Lightly flour your chopping board and turn out the dough onto the board. Knead the dough for approximately 3 minutes, until smooth and elastic (add more flour if dough is sticky), then cut into six balls of similar size. Add more flour to the chopping board, then flatten each ball with a rolling pin to make large, very thin circles — each flat bread should be about 20–22 cm (8–8½ in) in diameter. You will need to add more flour as you go along to ensure the flat bread does not stick and can be rolled out paper-thin.

Heat a large non-stick frying pan over medium–high heat and cook each flat bread for about 1 minute each side, or until bubbles appear and the bread becomes browned in spots. For soft wraps, don't cook them for too long. The longer they are left in the pan, the crunchier they will be.

Recipe by Bianca Rothwell.

Potato and Pesto Pizza

Serves 2, preparation time 20 minutes, cooking time 15 minutes
(plus additional time to make Spelt Flat Bread, Parsley Pesto and Caramelized Leek Sauce)

- 2–3 pieces Spelt Flat Bread (p. 155)
- 1 portion Parsley Pesto (p. 189)
- 3–4 white potatoes, peeled and finely sliced into discs
- Caramelized Leek Sauce (p. 130)
- quality sea salt, to taste
- ¼ cup finely chopped fresh chives
- handful of cashew nuts, chopped (optional)

Preheat the oven to 180°C (350°F). Insert a pizza stone into the oven before pre-heating or line a large flat baking tray with baking paper. Make the Spelt Flat Bread, Parsley Pesto and Caramelized Leek Sauce if not already prepared.

Place the flat breads onto the baking tray, spread with the pesto and add a thin layer of potato. Top with the leek sauce, adding dollops intermittently, and season with salt. Place the pizza in the oven and bake for about 15 minutes or until the potato is soft. Remove from the oven, top with chives and raw cashew nuts and serve.

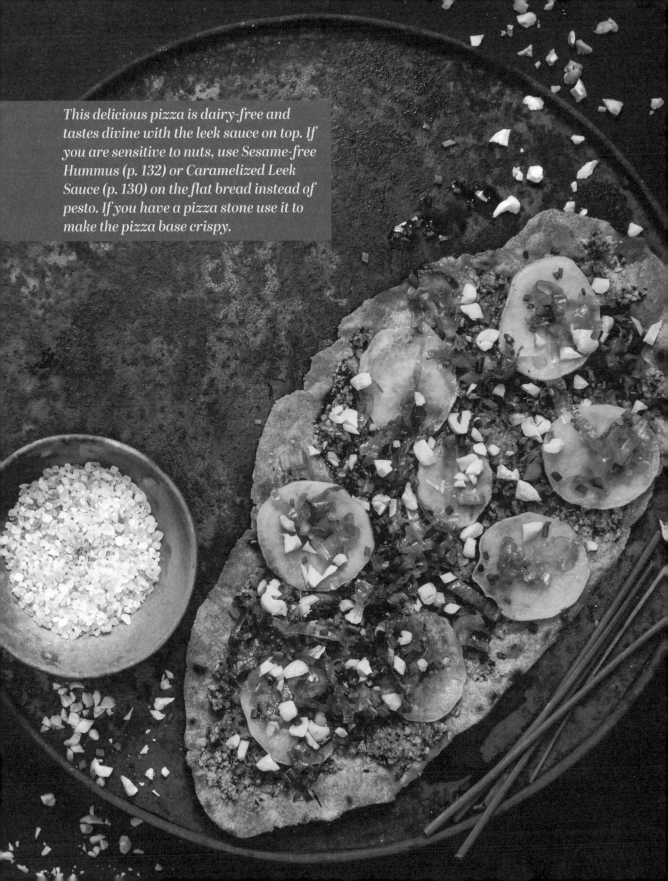

This delicious pizza is dairy-free and tastes divine with the leek sauce on top. If you are sensitive to nuts, use Sesame-free Hummus (p. 132) or Caramelized Leek Sauce (p. 130) on the flat bread instead of pesto. If you have a pizza stone use it to make the pizza base crispy.

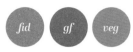

Design-your-own Sandwich

Serves 1, preparation time 5 minutes

Design your own sandwich using the following healthy breads (and gluten-free alternatives) and nutritious fillings.

Breads to choose from:
- spelt sourdough bread (store-bought — check ingredients)
- Spelt Flat Bread (p. 155)

Gluten-free alternatives:
- gluten-free bread (store-bought — check ingredients)
- plain rice cakes (no flavour enhancer, no additives, only salted)
- Mung Bean Sprout Pancakes (p. 168)

Spreads to choose from:
- Sesame-free Hummus (p. 132)
- Pink Pear Jam (p. 137)
- Bean Dip (p. 132)

Vegan sandwich fillings:
- leftover roast vegetables (peeled white potato, leeks, garlic, Brussels sprouts, swede/rutabaga) and Sesame-free Hummus (p. 132)
- Lentil Patties (p. 160), served with red cabbage, iceberg lettuce and Caramalized Leek Sauce (p. 130)
- Herbed Tofu Open Sandwich (p. 159)

Lean meat fillings (preferably organic or free-range):
- Bean Dip (p. 132) with iceberg lettuce, mung bean sprouts or shredded red cabbage and Caramalized Leek Sauce (p. 130) with cooked lamb, chicken or tofu.
- skinless cooked chicken (see notes) and mung bean sprouts
- fresh white fish such as flathead (flatfish), hake and dory fillets (not frozen, not leftovers)
- organic turkey breast (see notes)
- sliced lean roast lamb (home-cooked, no artificial additives)
- lamb steaks with fat removed
- roasted chicken (skinless), cooked with garlic and Parsley Oil (p. 134)

Notes:
- Only use organic or home-cooked meats as pre-sliced or deli turkey/lamb/chicken can contain irritating preservatives such as nitrates and flavour enhancers.
- These additional ingredients are only for those following the Eczema Detox Program: grated carrot, grated beetroot (beets), roasted sweet potato, roasted pumpkin (winter squash; occasionally, as pumpkin is high GI), snow peas/mangetout (not peas) and sliced banana.

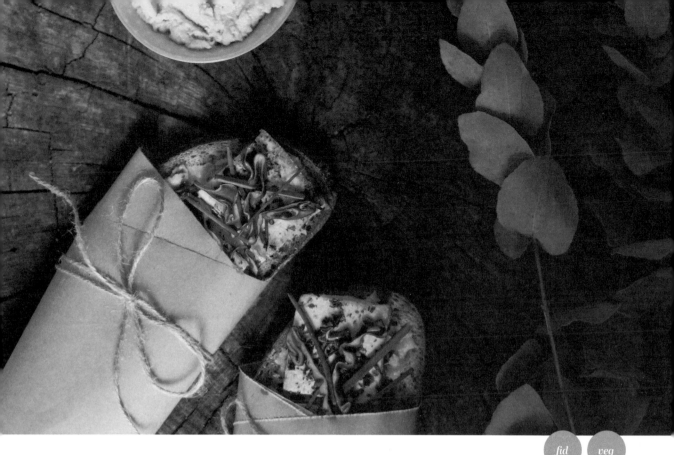

Herbed Tofu Open Sandwich

Serves 1, preparation time 5 minutes, cooking time 5 minutes

- spelt sourdough bread (store bought, wheat free)
- Sesame-free Hummus (p. 132)
- 3 x 1 cm (⅓ in) slices plain tofu (no additives, no flavourings)
- sprinkle of garlic powder
- sprinkle of quality sea salt
- fresh or dried chives
- Parsley Oil (p. 134)
- handful of red cabbage
- handful of iceberg lettuce

Season the tofu slices on each side with a sprinkle of garlic powder, salt and chives. Place a saucepan over medium heat and add a teaspoon of oil, then lightly fry the tofu, turning once until golden. Remove from the heat and drain on paper towels. Arrange the tofu, hummus, cabbage and iceberg lettuce onto the bread and serve.

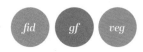

Lentil Patties

Makes 12 patties, preparation time 20 minutes, cooking time 20 minutes

- 3 medium-sized potatoes, peeled and cubed
- 2 medium stalks celery, halved lengthways and finely sliced
- 1 x 400 g (14 oz) can brown lentils, rinsed and drained well
- ¼ cup thinly sliced fresh chives
- ½ teaspoon quality sea salt (or to taste)
- 1 cup thinly sliced and diced red cabbage
- 1 serving of Egg Replacer (p. 211)
- 1 cup brown rice flour, plus extra for dusting
- Parsley Oil, for frying (p. 134)

Bring a saucepan of water to boil, add the potato and boil for 2 minutes. (Alternatively, if you have extra time you can steam the vegetables.) Add the celery and cook until all the vegetables are soft (about 3 minutes). Drain well, then place the vegetables into a blender or food processor and blend on low speed. Do not over-blend — the mixture should resemble a thick, chunky mash rather than a soup.

Add the mash to a large bowl, then add the lentils, chives, salt and cabbage. Mix the ingredients together then stir in the Egg Replacer (if using) and the flour until a sticky mixture has formed, adding more flour if the mixture is too wet.

Sprinkle some extra flour on a chopping board, then with your hands form the patties (not too thick: roughly 1 cm/⅓ in thick and a diameter of about 7 cm/2½ in). Then coat each side in the flour on the chopping board.

Place a large non-stick frying pan on medium heat (not high, as you will burn the oil), lightly coat in oil and cook the patties for about 3–5 minutes on each side or until golden on each side. (Cook the patties until they become firm and cooked through. Turn down the heat if they are browning too quickly.) Remove from the pan and place onto paper towels to drain the oil.
Recipe by Katie Layland.

Note: you can enjoy these patties freshly cooked or refrigerate or freeze them for later use. Reheat frozen patties in the oven on a lined baking tray at 180°C (350°F) for about 10 minutes or until warmed through (or lightly fry them in a non-stick frying pan).

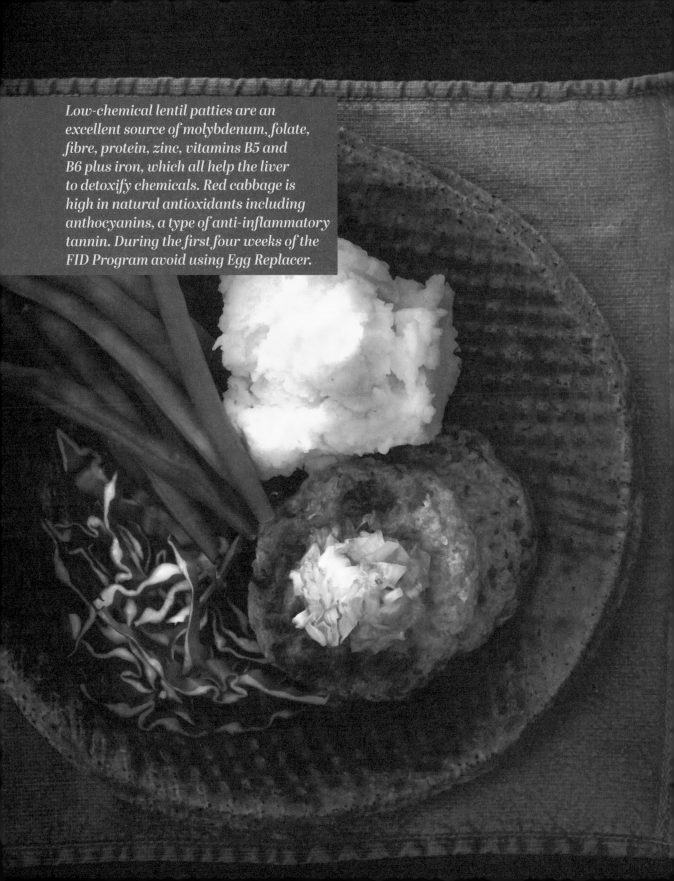

Low-chemical lentil patties are an excellent source of molybdenum, folate, fibre, protein, zinc, vitamins B5 and B6 plus iron, which all help the liver to detoxify chemicals. Red cabbage is high in natural antioxidants including anthocyanins, a type of anti-inflammatory tannin. During the first four weeks of the FID Program avoid using Egg Replacer.

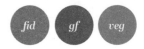

Mashed Potato

Serves 2, preparation time 10 minutes, cooking time 10 minutes

Potatoes are the most underrated food of our time. They are not trendy but they are incredibly nutritious and an excellent source of vitamin C. Potatoes are an alkalizing vegetable and a rich source of vitamin B6, potassium and copper for healthy skin. Peeled white potatoes are also low in salicylates. Choose gluten-free milk if necessary.

- 4 white potatoes, thickly peeled and cubed
- ¼ cup rice milk, oat milk or organic soy milk
- ¼ teaspoon quality sea salt, or to taste
- ½ teaspoon garlic powder
- 1 tablespoon finely chopped fresh chives or parsley

Add plenty of water to a saucepan, then bring to the boil and add the potatoes. Cook for about 10 minutes or until soft. When nice and soft, drain the potatoes and place them back in the saucepan. Add the rice milk, salt and garlic powder and mash until creamy. Add the herbs, mix and serve.

Note: refer to potato information in the FID food shopping list on p. 78.

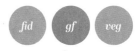

New Potato and Leek Soup

Serves 6–8, preparation time 20 minutes, cooking time 20 minutes

Potatoes are a rich source of antioxidants and vitamin B6, and a good source of vitamin C, potassium, copper, manganese, vitamin B5 and dietary fibre for healthy bowels and clear skin. Leeks contain magnesium, vitamin K, folate and other B-group vitamins, plus a powerful cancer-fighting flavonol called kaempferol which has anti-inflammatory and anti-fungal properties.

- 1 teaspoon Parsley Oil (p. 134)
- 1 large leek, green parts removed, white part washed and finely sliced
- 2 large cloves garlic, minced
- 5 cups filtered water
- 1.2 kg+ (2½ lbs) white potatoes (see note)
- 1 cup dried red lentils
- 2 Brussels sprouts, finely sliced
- ¾–1 teaspoon quality sea salt (or to taste)
- fresh chives, to serve

In a stockpot or very large saucepan, heat a splash of oil on medium heat and lightly fry the leek and garlic. Turn up the heat and add the water, then cover and bring to the boil.

Meanwhile, peel and dice the potatoes and add them to the saucepan. Then prepare the dried lentils by rinsing them thoroughly in a bowl of water, straining them and removing any discoloured ones. Add them to the saucepan along with the Brussels sprouts. Cover and bring to the boil. Reduce the heat to low and simmer for 20–30 minutes, stirring occasionally. Stir in the salt the remove soup from the heat and allow to cool for a few minutes.

One batch at a time, process the soup in a blender or food processor until smooth. If the soup is too thick, add water boiled from the kettle (you will most likely need 1–2 cups extra). Serve garnished with freshly chopped chives.

Note: buy only white potatoes and they must be peeled in order to be salicylate-free.
Read potato information in FID food shopping list on p.78.

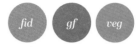

Lentil Vegie Soup

Serves 4, preparation time 10 minutes, cooking time 18 minutes

- 1 large leek, green part removed
- 1 teaspoon Parsley Oil (p. 134) or filtered water
- 3 stalks celery, finely sliced
- 2 medium white potatoes, peeled and diced (see notes)
- 1½ cups dried red lentils, rinsed and discoloured ones removed
- 6 cups filtered water (or Alkaline Vegetable Broth, p. 167)
- ½ teaspoon garlic powder
- 2 tablespoons finely diced chives or parsley stems, plus extra to serve
- ¾ teaspoon quality sea salt (or to taste)

Wash the leek, removing any dirt in the layers, then halve it lengthways and finely slice the white/pale green part. Place a medium–large saucepan on medium heat and add the oil (or water for oil-free cooking) and sauté the leek for 3 minutes or until soft. Then add the celery, potato, lentils, water and garlic powder and bring to the boil. Turn the heat down to low, place on the lid and simmer for 15 minutes or until the lentils and vegetables are soft (but not overcooked). Add the chives and salt, stir and remove from the heat. Serve in bowls and garnish with finely sliced chives.

Recipe by Katie Layland.

Notes:

- If you are following the Eczema Detox Program you can add two medium carrots, finely diced.
- Red split lentils work best in the recipe, but if using dried brown lentils simmer for 25 minutes or until soft.

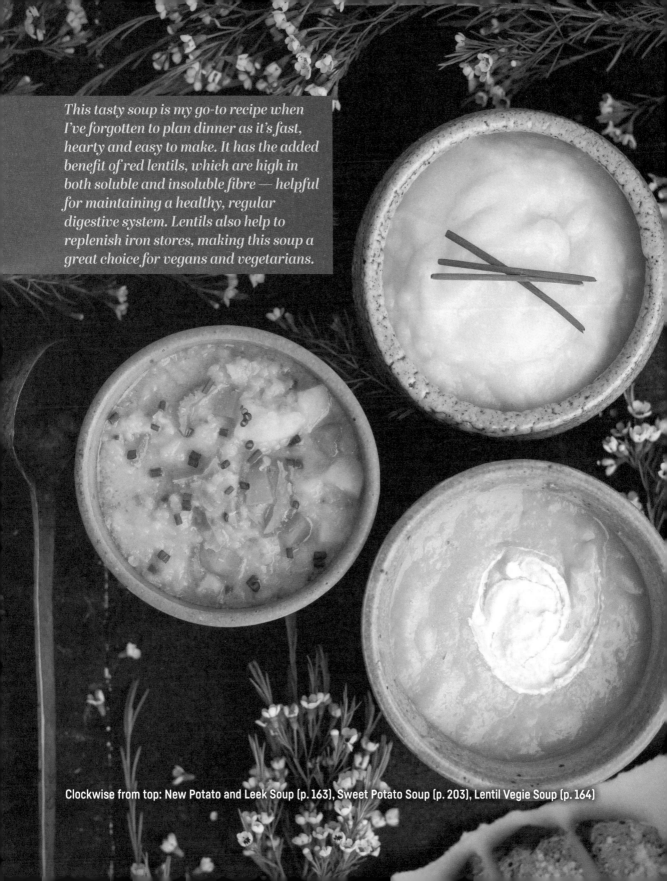

This tasty soup is my go-to recipe when I've forgotten to plan dinner as it's fast, hearty and easy to make. It has the added benefit of red lentils, which are high in both soluble and insoluble fibre — helpful for maintaining a healthy, regular digestive system. Lentils also help to replenish iron stores, making this soup a great choice for vegans and vegetarians.

Clockwise from top: New Potato and Leek Soup (p. 163), Sweet Potato Soup (p. 203), Lentil Vegie Soup (p. 164)

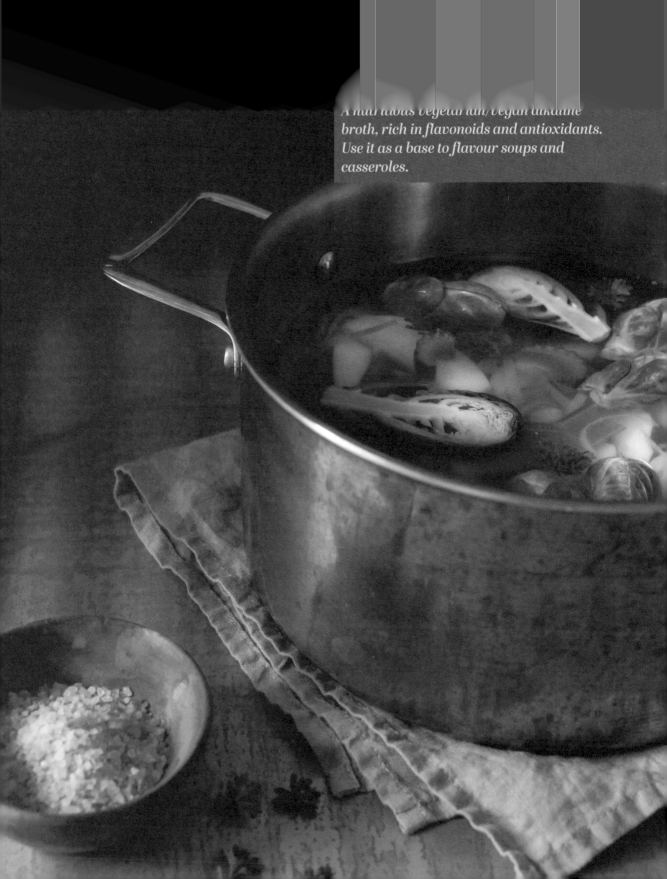

A nutritious vegetarian/vegan alkaline broth, rich in flavonoids and antioxidants. Use it as a base to flavour soups and casseroles.

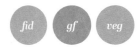

Alkaline Vegetable Broth

Serves 4, preparation time 10 minutes, cooking time 1 hour

- ½ leek, finely sliced
- 2 cloves garlic, minced
- 3 stalks celery, chopped
- 3 Brussels sprouts, chopped
- 3 white potatoes, peeled thickly and diced (see notes)
- 1 tablespoon parsley
- 5 litres filtered water
- ½–¾ teaspoon quality sea salt (or to taste)

Wash the leek and remove any dirt in the layers. In a stockpot or very large saucepan, heat a splash of filtered water on medium heat and lightly sauté the leek and garlic for 5 minutes. Then add all the remaining ingredients to the saucepan, cover and bring to the boil. Reduce the heat to low and simmer for 1 hour, stirring occasionally. Remove from the heat and allow to cool for a few minutes.

Strain the broth, pressing out the liquid from the vegetables using a spatula or the base of a cup. Remove the vegetables and keep the liquid.

Notes:
- Broth will last for a week if refrigerated. Store the leftover broth in clean glass jars or containers, and freeze the leftovers.
- If you are following the Eczema Detox Program you can add 1 large diced carrot.
- Buy only white potatoes and they must be peeled in order to be salicylate-free. Read potato information in the FID food shopping list on p. 78.

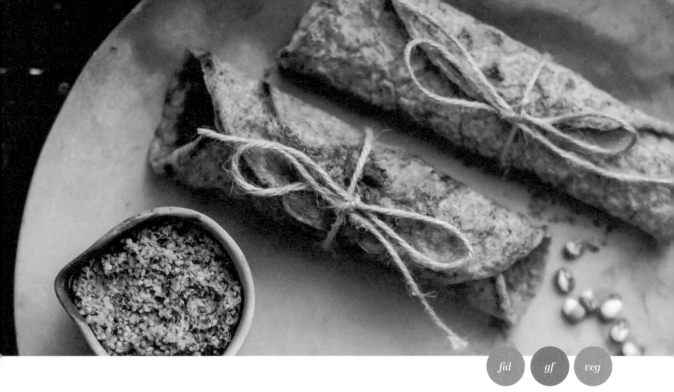

fid *gf* *veg*

Mung Bean Sprout Pancakes

Makes 6 small pancakes, preparation time 5 minutes, cooking time 15 minutes

- 200 g (7 oz) mung bean sprouts
- ¾ cup filtered water or more for thinner consistency
- ½ teaspoon quality sea salt, or to taste
- 2 tablespoons arrowroot flour (or eczema-friendly flour of choice)
- Parsley Oil (p. 134), for frying

Rinse the mung bean sprouts, drain well, then place into a blender with the water and salt. Blend on medium–high speed until it is almost a smooth consistency. The consistency should be that of a thin pancake so slowly add extra water until you reach this. Add the flour and blend again until smooth.

Place a frying pan over medium heat and drizzle in a little oil. When the pan is ready, add about ¼ cup of the pancake mixture, swirling the pan slightly if you want thinner pancakes. When browned on one side flip and cook until slightly brown on both sides. Repeat the process.

Serve warm. Store leftovers in the refrigerator and reheat before serving.
Recipe by Katie Layland.

Sprouting mung beans

Mung bean sprouts are one of the few strongly alkalizing foods available so they are fantastic for your skin. They contain magnesium, vitamin K, folate, potassium and vitamin C and they are salicylate-free. Mung bean sprouts need to be rinsed before use and if you can't find them at your local supermarket it's easy to sprout your own. Don't get them mixed up with bean sprouts — refer to the photo on p. 51.

You can use this method to sprout mung beans, barley or lentils — these are your eczema-safe choices for sprouting but mung beans are the easiest to sprout. If using lentils they must not be 'split' lentils as they won't sprout. Any bean that is split or broken will not sprout, so remove these as they will remain hard.

· ⅓ cup dried mung beans
· wide glass jar or container
· cheesecloth or mesh
· elastic band
· filtered water

Wash the mung beans before use and remove the damaged ones that look darker or split. After rinsing them, place them into the glass jar or container. Fill the jar with lukewarm water to help soften any hard beans and cover the jar with a piece of breathable cloth or mesh, then secure with an elastic band. Set aside on the kitchen bench in low light, away from direct sunlight and not in a dark cupboard. Soak them overnight.

The next morning, drain off the excess water and rinse the beans with water. To make the rinsing process simple, keep the beans in the jar and keep the mesh on and rinse. If using cloth, remove the cloth, keep the beans in the jar, fill the jar with water and place a mesh strainer over the top and drain the water. You will need to rinse and drain twice a day for about two to three days (shorter time in hot weather, longer in cold weather).

As soon as the beans have sprouted, drain any excess water, dry the sprouts and store them in the refrigerator, wrapped in a paper towel (or something to soak up the excess moisture) in an airtight container. Use them within four days for maximum freshness.

Lamb and Sticky Leeks

Serves 2, preparation time 15 minutes, cooking time 15 minutes

Lamb is a rich source of iron and protein, and when combined with highly alkalizing leeks and red cabbage creates a nutritious acid–alkaline balanced meal.

- Caramelized Leek Sauce (p. 130)
- ½ cup white or brown rice
  (not jasmine or basmati)
- 2–4 lean lamb steaks
  (depending on appetite and size of steaks)
- Parsley Oil (p. 134)
- quality sea salt, to taste
- garlic powder (optional), to taste
- 1 cup green beans, ends trimmed
- 1 cup finely chopped red cabbage

Make the Caramelized Leek Sauce and set aside. Preheat the grill (broiler) to a medium–high heat.

Place the rice into a saucepan with plenty of water, then bring to the boil and cook according to packet instructions. Drain, cover and set aside.

Coat the lamb with the oil and sprinkle on the salt and garlic powder, if desired. When the grill is hot, cook the lamb for about 6 minutes each side, turning once, until the outside is browned and the inside is slightly pink.

Meanwhile, using a non-stick frying pan and 1 tablespoon of filtered water, lightly sauté the red cabbage and green beans on medium–high heat for 1–2 minutes. Transfer the vegetables to a plate and serve with the rice and lamb topped with Caramelized Leek Sauce.

San Choy Bau

Serves 2, preparation time 15 minutes, cooking time 20 minutes

You will love this tasty low-chemical version of the classic Chinese favourite. It has a lovely blend of alkaline vegetables and iron-rich mince (or beans to make it vegan). Instead of organic lamb mince you can use chicken or turkey mince, tofu or black beans.

- 2 teaspoons Parsley Oil (p. 134)
- 1 large leek, white part only, washed and finely sliced
- ½ cup finely shredded red cabbage
- 2 stalks celery, halved lengthways and finely diced
- 500 g (1 lb) preservative-free organic lamb mince or 2 cups cooked black beans
- 2 cloves garlic, peeled and minced
- 1 tablespoon dried or fresh chives or parsley
- ½ cup filtered water
- quality sea salt, to taste
- 4–6 large, whole iceberg lettuce leaves, to serve
- mung bean sprouts (optional)
- Maple Dressing (optional, p. 135)

If you are cooking black beans, see below for cooking instructions (use 1 cup of dried black beans or 1 x 400 g (14 oz) can of beans).

Heat 1 teaspoon of oil in a medium-sized saucepan on medium heat, add the leek and sauté for about 2 minutes. Then add the cabbage and celery and cook for around 2 minutes, until tender but still crisp. Remove from the saucepan and set aside.

Using the same saucepan, add 1 teaspoon of oil, the mince (or beans), garlic and chives, breaking the mince apart to prevent lumps. Briefly cook on high heat, stirring occasionally, until the mince has separated and browned. Add the water and salt, reduce the heat to low and cover and cook for 10 minutes or until the water has evaporated.

Place the lettuce leaves on plates and fill with the mince or beans. Top with the cabbage, leeks and mung bean sprouts. Drizzle on a teaspoon of Maple Dressing, if desired.
Recipe by Deb Wiseman.

How to cook dried beans and chickpeas

Rinse the beans and remove any stones. Place the beans into a large saucepan, cover with water (about 7 cm/3 in above the beans) and soak for about 8 hours or overnight. If the weather is hot, place in the refrigerator so they do not ferment. Drain and rinse the beans, return them to the saucepan and cover with fresh water. Bring to the boil then simmer on low heat for 30–40 minutes. Drain and rinse.

Steamed Fish Parcels with Mashed Potato

Serves 2, preparation time 10 minutes, cooking time 25 minutes

- 1 portion Mashed Potato (p. 162)
- 2 fresh flathead fillets (or other fresh white fleshed fish)
- Parsley Oil (p. 134)
- sprinkle of garlic powder
- sprinkle of quality sea salt
- handful flat-leaf parsley, washed and chopped, stems removed
- 1 tablespoon filtered water or Alkaline Vegetable Broth (p. 167)
- 2 spring onions (shallots, scallions), sliced
- 2 handfuls green beans
- ½ cup finely shredded red cabbage
- Optional: cut 1 garlic bulb in half (see photo), drizzle on a little oil and roast on a baking tray for 15-20 minutes, then place it on top of the cooked fish before serving.

Preheat the oven to 200°C (400°F). Make the Mashed Potato if not already prepared.

Next, tear off two sheets of aluminum foil each about 25 x 15 cm (10 x 6 in; they should be big enough to wrap the fish). Then place baking paper of the same size over the top of each sheet of foil. Place the fish onto the paper, then drizzle with the oil and sprinkle on the garlic powder, salt and parsley. Fold the paper and foil over the fish, folding the edges of the foil several times to seal in the steam and leaving one edge open. Gently pour the water or broth into the parcels through the open edge, fold over the remaining edge so that the parcel is completely sealed.

Place the parcels onto a baking tray, then place in the oven. Cook until the parcels puff up (about 10 minutes on average, depending on the thickness of the fish fillets). Do not overcook. Remove from the oven and open the parcel along centre to reveal the fish and let the steam escape so the fish does not overcook. (be careful not to get burned by the release of steam). Serve from the opened foil package.

Meanwhile, place a small frying pan over high heat and lightly fry the spring onions, green beans and red cabbage for about 5 minutes. Season with salt.

Serve the fish with the vegetables and a side of Mashed Potato.

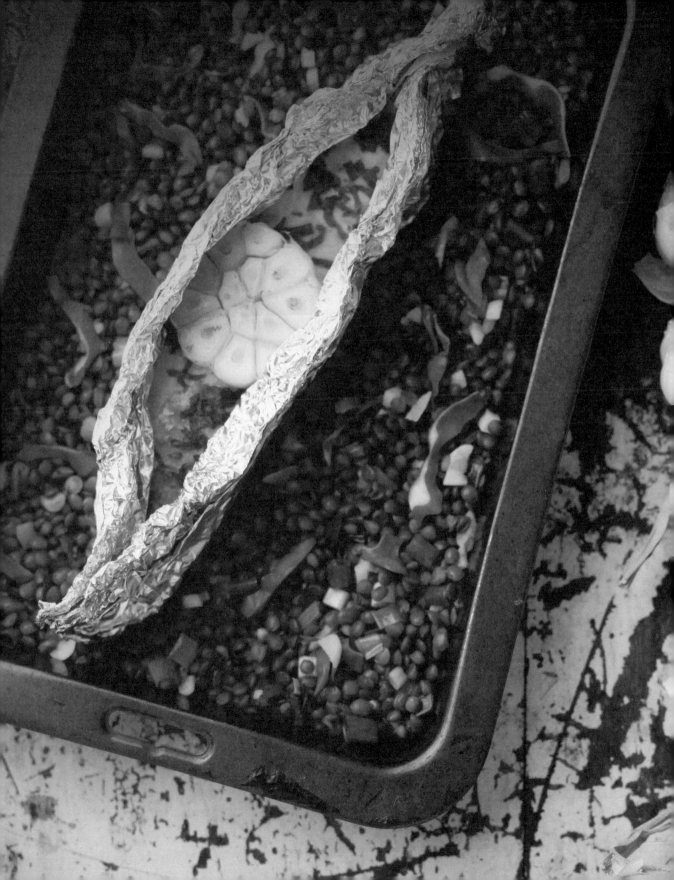

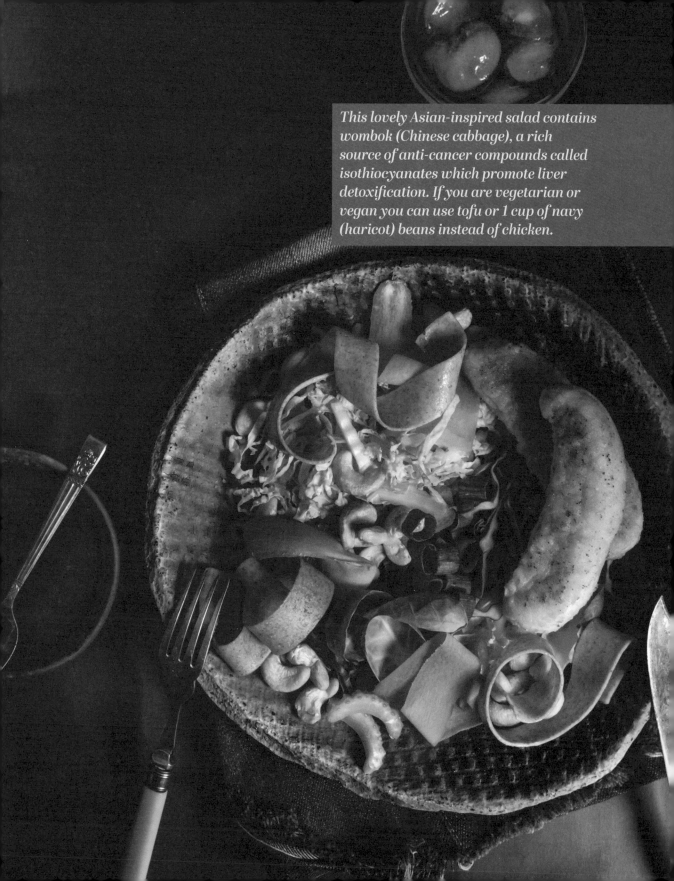

This lovely Asian-inspired salad contains wombok (Chinese cabbage), a rich source of anti-cancer compounds called isothiocyanates which promote liver detoxification. If you are vegetarian or vegan you can use tofu or 1 cup of navy (haricot) beans instead of chicken.

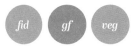

Wombok Noodle Salad

Serves 2, preparation time 15 minutes, cooking time 15 minutes

- Maple Dressing (p. 135), to serve
- 4 large skinless chicken tenderloins (or 1 packet plain tofu)
- sprinkle of garlic powder
- sprinkle of quality sea salt
- 2 tablespoons chickpea (besan, gram) flour (or rice flour) (optional)
- 1 tablespoon Parsley Oil (p. 134)
- 4 spring onions (shallots, scallions), washed and thinly sliced
- ½ white wombok/Chinese cabbage (about 2 cups), washed and shredded
- 1 stalk celery, washed and finely sliced
- 200 g (7 oz) dried rice noodles (see notes)
- ½ cup raw cashews (optional)

Make the Maple Dressing and store it in a jar.

Dice the chicken (or tofu) and place it into a sealable plastic bag, along with the garlic powder, salt and chickpea flour, then seal the bag and shake it until the chicken is coated (alternatively, use a bowl to combine the ingredients and push chicken pieces into the mixture on all sides). Place a large frying pan over medium heat, then add the oil and cook the chicken/tofu until golden and cooked through. Remove from the heat and place the chicken/tofu onto paper towels to drain.

Place the spring onions, Chinese cabbage and celery into a large bowl. Prepare the noodles according to the packet instructions, then add the chicken, cashews and noodles to the salad and toss gently to combine.

Shake the Maple Dressing to combine the ingredients and add to the salad just before serving (about 1 tablespoon of dressing per person, or more if desired), and lightly mix through.

Notes:
- Wombok/Chinese cabbage contains moderate salicylates so if you are following the FID Program use red cabbage for the first three weeks.
- Avoid cashews if you are following the FID Program or are allergic to them.
- When choosing rice noodles, ensure they are gluten free if you are gluten intolerant.
- You can substitute spelt pasta if you are not gluten intolerant (see photo).

Crispy Chicken Pasta

Serves 1, preparation time 20 minutes, cooking time 15 minutes

- 1 cup gluten-free pasta (or mung bean pasta or spelt pasta if not sensitive to gluten)
- 2 chicken tenderloins or 1 chicken thigh fillet, fat removed
- 2 tablespoons chickpea (besan, gram) flour (or brown rice flour)
- 1 teaspoon dried parsley or chives
- sprinkle of quality sea salt
- handful of green beans, ends trimmed
- ¼ cup finely shredded red cabbage
- Parsley Oil (p. 134), for frying
- 1–2 teaspoons rice malt syrup (brown rice syrup) or real maple syrup (optional)

Bring a large saucepan of water to the boil and add the pasta. Cook according to the packet instructions. Drain and set aside.

Chop the chicken into bite-sized pieces, removing any strings or fat. Place the flour, dried herbs and salt into a sealable plastic sandwich bag, then add the chicken, seal the bag and shake until the chicken is coated (alternatively, use a bowl to combine the ingredients and push chicken pieces into the mixture on all sides).

Heat a large non-stick frying pan over medium heat, add a little oil and cook the chicken until crispy on the outside and cooked through (about 7–10 minutes, depending on the size of the pieces). Remove from the heat and place onto paper towels to drain the oil.

Wipe the frying pan then place back on medium heat, add 1 teaspoon of oil and lightly sauté the beans and red cabbage with 1 teaspoon of syrup. If the pasta needs refreshing before serving, run some boiling water over the top, drain and serve with the sweet vegetables on top and chicken on the side.

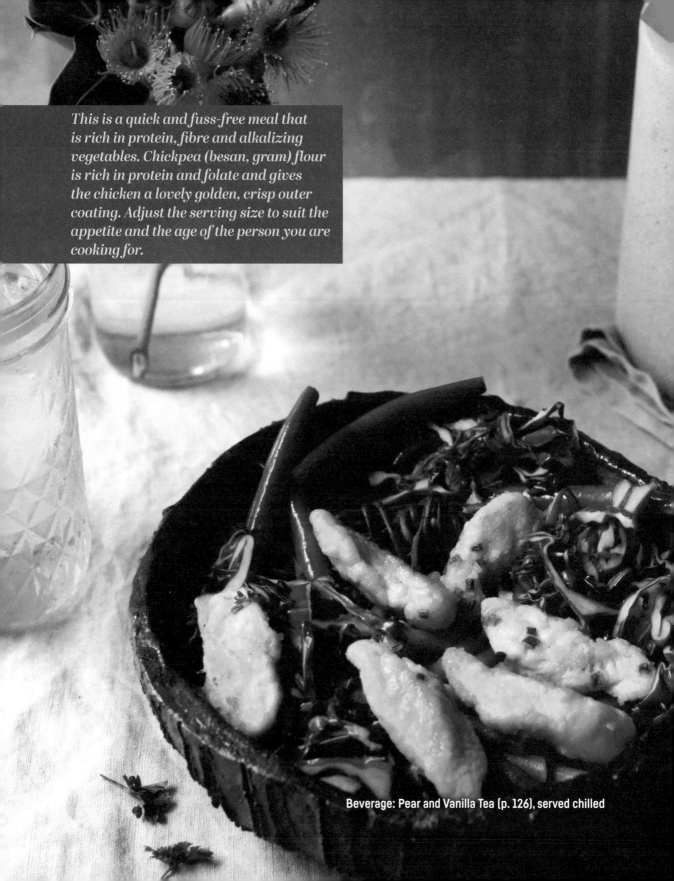

This is a quick and fuss-free meal that is rich in protein, fibre and alkalizing vegetables. Chickpea (besan, gram) flour is rich in protein and folate and gives the chicken a lovely golden, crisp outer coating. Adjust the serving size to suit the appetite and the age of the person you are cooking for.

Beverage: Pear and Vanilla Tea (p. 126), served chilled

Desserts

These low-salicylate desserts are treats you can enjoy while on the diet. As this is ultimately a healing program, do not overindulge: the recipes use natural syrups in lesser amounts than regular desserts but any sweetener is still classed as sugar. Calcium powder is often added for acid–alkaline balance and nutritional benefits.

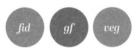

Pear Crumble

Serves 7–8, preparation time 20 minutes, cooking time 20–30 minutes

- 10 ripe pears, peeled and core removed (see note for alternative)
- ¼ cup filtered water or Electrolyte Pear Juice (p. 128)

Topping:

- 2 cups rolled oats (use gluten-free if possible)
- 1 cup quinoa flakes
- ¼ cup flaxseeds/linseeds (if you have tested flaxseeds in week 3 of the FID Program)
- ¼ cup real maple syrup (or ½ cup rice malt syrup)
- 1½ tablespoons Parsley Oil (p. 134)

Preheat the oven to 180°C (350°F) and line a large baking dish (e.g. 22 cm/8½ in round dish) with baking paper, or oil the sides with oil. Slice the pears and arrange them in the dish. Sprinkle the water or Electrolyte Pear Juice over the pears.

In a large bowl, combine the oats, quinoa flakes, flaxseeds, syrup and oil and mix until crumbly and sticky. If the mixture is too dry, add more syrup. Spread the crumble evenly over the pears. Place in the oven and bake for 20–30 minutes, checking often, until the pears are stewing and soft and the topping is lightly golden.

Notes:

- Avoid Nashi/Asian and Ya pears (apple-shaped pears) as they contain salicylates.
- If you do not have fresh pear, use 2 x 400 g/14 oz cans of pears in sugar syrup, drained (avoid corn syrup and avoid pears in juice as they are rich in salicylates).

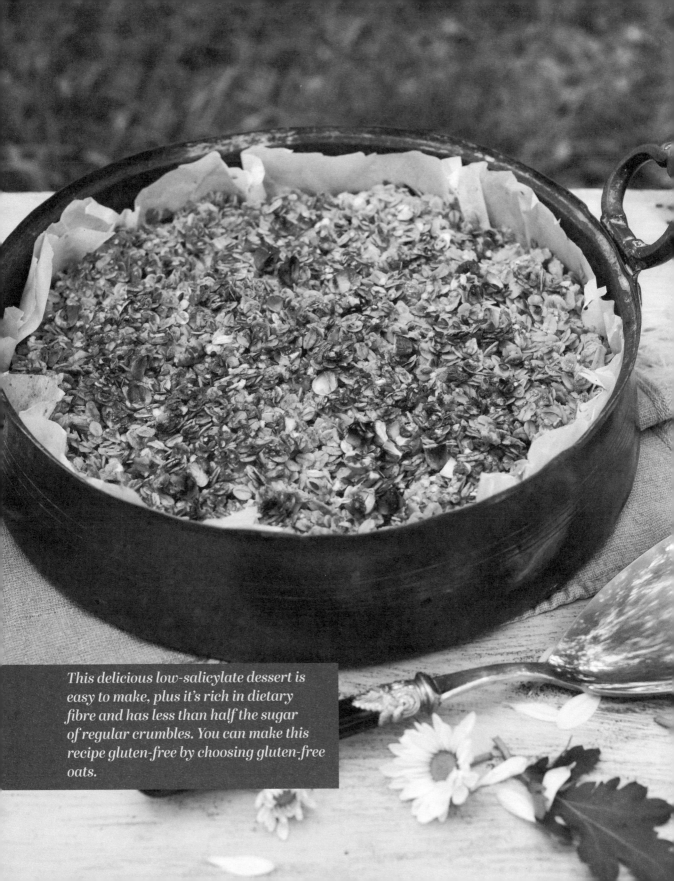

This delicious low-salicylate dessert is easy to make, plus it's rich in dietary fibre and has less than half the sugar of regular crumbles. You can make this recipe gluten-free by choosing gluten-free oats.

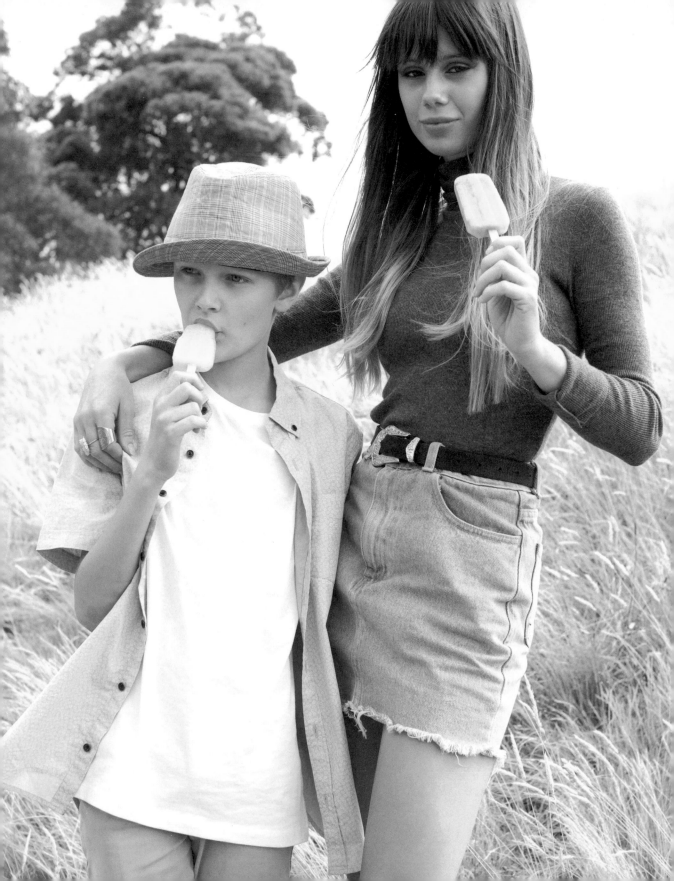

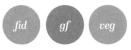

Pear Sorbet

Serves 2, preparation time 5 minutes, cooking time 5 minutes (plus overnight freezing time)

The humble pear is an incredibly healthy fruit, rich in two types of fibre for bowel health, plus anti-inflammatory nutrients including quercetin and vitamin C. The addition of calcium powder makes this an acid–alkaline balanced dessert (and it's a fun way to have your calcium).

- 4–5 ripe pears, peeled (avoid Asian/Nashi or Ya pears) (or 1 x 400 g/14 oz can pears in syrup, drained)
- 3 g (3 scoops) fine calcium powder (optional, see 'Useful resources', p. 220)
- filtered water
- real maple syrup, to taste (optional, if using fresh pears)

If using canned pears, be sure to avoid any containing corn syrup. Drain and discard the sugar syrup. Cut the pears into small pieces. If using fresh pears, fill a medium-sized saucepan with water, then add the pears and bring to the boil, cooking until the pears are soft (about 5 minutes). Strain the pears and refrigerate the liquid for later use (as a cold drink or in Pear and Vanilla Tea, p. 126). Allow the pears to cool.

Place the pear pieces into a freezer bag or large freezer-proof containers. Freeze the pears flat so that you can easily break off pieces when frozen. Leave in the freezer for at least 3 hours, or until frozen.

Place the frozen chunks of pear into a food processor and a splash of pear water to help it blend, and blend on medium speed until smooth. If using fresh pears do a taste test and add maple syrup if desired. The consistency should be like sorbet or soft serve ice-cream. Serve immediately. Freeze leftovers in ice block trays.

Notes:
- Optional: add approx. five strands of saffron to colour and flavour the pears during the pear boiling stage (or to colour and flavour the ice blocks, as shown in the photo).
- To make the ice blocks (ice lollies/popsicles) pour the mixture into ice block moulds and freeze until firm.

fid   veg

New Anzac Cookies

Makes 20 biscuits, preparation time 15 minutes, cooking time 20 minutes

This recipe is an eczema-friendly take on an Australian classic. These sweet Anzac biscuits contain less sugar and more wholemeal goodness than the conventional type, and they're butter- and dairy-free. Although this recipe is wheat-free, it's not suitable if you have a wheat allergy or gluten intolerance as spelt contains gluten. You can use an alternative flour if desired (check the FID food shopping list on p. 78 for choices).

- 1½ cups rolled oats
- 1 cup wholemeal plain spelt flour
- ⅔ cup maple sugar (see note)
- ½ cup Parsley Oil (p. 134) or rice bran oil
- 1 tablespoon real maple syrup
- 1 teaspoon bicarbonate of soda (baking soda)
- 1–2 tablespoons filtered water (optional)

Preheat the oven to 150°C (300°F). Line two baking trays with baking paper. In a mixing bowl, combine the oats, spelt flour and maple sugar. Place a small saucepan over high heat, then add the oil and maple syrup and heat and mix until the syrup begins to bubble (ensure it does not burn). Promptly add the bicarbonate of soda and mix with a spoon until it foams. Quickly remove the saucepan from the heat and pour the hot foaming liquid onto the dry ingredients and mix well. The cookie dough should be slightly wet and stick when pressed into shape. If the mixture is too dry, add 1 or 2 tablespoons of water and mix.

Using a dessert spoon and your hands, form the dough into approximately 20 small balls (about 2 cm/1 in wide) then place them on the trays and flatten slightly (they will expand so allow room between the cookies). Bake for 15 minutes or until golden brown.

Note: if you cannot find maple sugar use organic white sugar (ideally only for special occasions such as birthdays, as sugar is highly acid-forming and not good for eczema). Raw sugar contains salicylates.

Chapter 14
Recipes: Eczema Detox Program

The recipes in this chapter are for those following the Eczema Detox Program, and have been specially crafted to cleanse the body and heal your skin from the inside out. This section includes recipes containing *moderate* levels of natural chemicals, which are denoted with an 's' for moderate salicylates or 'a' for moderate amines. If an ingredient contains high levels of salicylates or amines you will see 'ss' or 'aa' beside the ingredient.

If you are following the FID Program the goal is to become *less* sensitive to chemicals over time and progress to the Detox recipes in this chapter once you pass the salicylate and/ or amine tests detailed in Chapter 10. If you have a young child with eczema, ideally begin with the FID Program recipes (starting on p. 124) and modify the recipes to suit your child's age, allergies and eating abilities. Then progress to the Detox recipes in this chapter once your child's eczema has improved.

Skin Friend

If you want to give your juices and smoothies an extra skin detoxification vitamin boost, you can add Skin Friend AM and PM (available at www.skinfriend.com). Simply add them to your prepared juice or smoothie, or consume them mixed into filtered water and taken with a meal. For the correct Skin Friend dosage, refer to the packaging.

More recipes

If you are following the Eczema Detox Program you can try any recipe in this book, even the ones labelled 'fid' (in the previous chapter).

Drinks

Hydrate your skin from the inside out and boost liver detoxification with the following detox drinks:

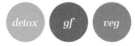

Cashew Nut Milk

Makes 4 cups, preparation time 5 minutes (plus 4+ hours soaking time)

Make your own creamy nut milk — this one is both low in salicylates and rich in alkalizing calcium so it's acid–alkaline balanced.

- 1 cup raw cashews (must not be roasted or salted)
- filtered water, for soaking (enough to cover)
- 3 cups filtered water
- 5 g (5 scoops) fine calcium powder

Place the cashews in a container, cover them with water and a lid and place them away from direct light. Allow the cashews to soak for at least 4 hours or overnight.

Drain and rinse the cashews (they must be rinsed to remove any residue), then place them into a high-powdered blender (in batches if necessary) with the filtered water and calcium powder, and blend until smooth. Pour into a jug, cover and refrigerate. Note it is best to avoid adding sweetener while on the Eczema Detox Program — try to wean yourself off sweetener — but you can add some rice malt syrup if needed.

Notes:
- If using a high-powered blender make the milk in two batches. If using a regular blender the milk might need straining (I recommend switching to a high-powered blender, the type made specifically for smoothies … you'll never go back).
- Allergy testing can be inaccurate so you might not know if you are sensitive to cashews. If your tests show you are allergic to cashews, avoid them. If you are unsure, test cashews during the FID Program (see instructions on p. 84).

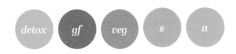

Healthy Skin Smoothie

Serves 1 adult, preparation time 5 minutes (plus optional freezing time)

This drink is designed to hydrate your skin and boost liver detoxification. Pre-freeze a peeled banana to make a cold smoothie. Adding pure pea protein powder or rice protein powder (or a combination of both) helps to strengthen your hair, skin and nails. Choose between banana and papaya or use both.

- ½ ripe banana, chopped (a)
  (use fresh or frozen peeled banana)
- 1 slice papaya or pawpaw, skin removed (a)
  (use fresh or frozen)
- 1½ cups milk of choice (see notes)
- ½ teaspoon flaxseed oil (sa)
- 2 tablespoons pea/rice protein powder
  (optional; no flavourings)
- Skin Friend (optional)

Combine all the ingredients in a high-powered blender and blend on high until smooth.

Notes:
- If pre-freezing the banana, peel it first, slice it into bite-sized pieces, then store in a freezer bag or sealed container. Use within three to four days.
- You can add 1 sprig of parsley, finely chopped (for alkalizing).
- Milk options: Cashew Nut Milk (p. 184), organic gluten-free soy milk, rice milk or oat milk.
- If you are sensitive to glutamates/MSG do not consume any type of protein powder.

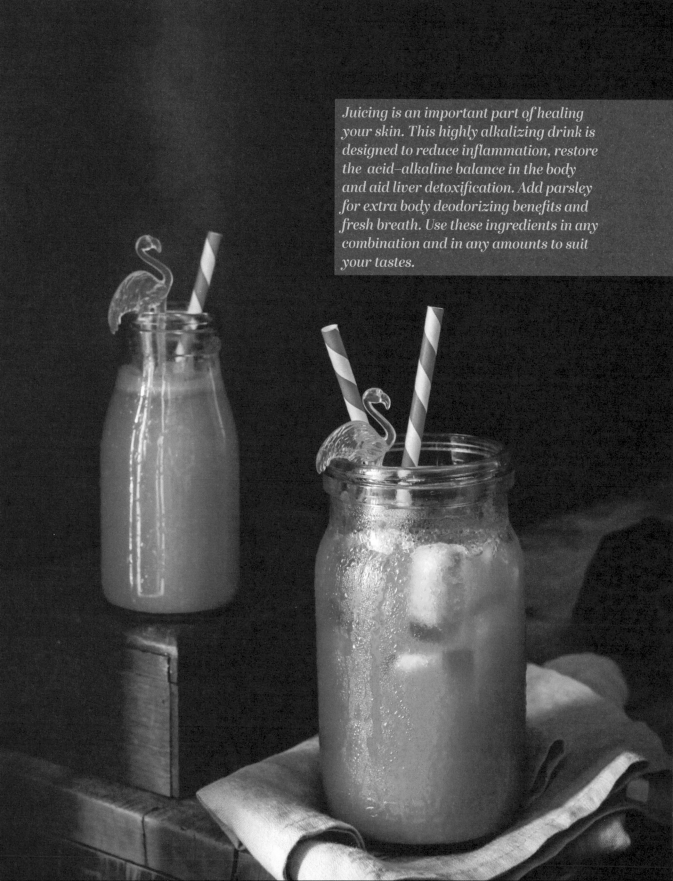

Juicing is an important part of healing your skin. This highly alkalizing drink is designed to reduce inflammation, restore the acid–alkaline balance in the body and aid liver detoxification. Add parsley for extra body deodorizing benefits and fresh breath. Use these ingredients in any combination and in any amounts to suit your tastes.

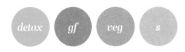

Healthy Skin Juice

Serves 2 or 2 days' supply for 1 adult, preparation time 5 minutes

Choose from the following:

- 4 stalks celery
- 2 peeled pears (must be ripe; avoid Asian/ Nashi or Ya pears) (s: the skin contains salicylates)
- 2 carrots, tops removed (s)
- ¼ small beetroot (beet), scrubbed (s)
- 1 cup iceberg lettuce
- ½ cup red cabbage
- handful of fresh parsley
- ½ cup fresh mung bean sprouts, rinsed
- Skin Friend AM (optional)

Wash and scrub the chosen vegetables and pears. Using a juicing machine, juice the fruits and vegetables, ending by adding a splash of filtered water.

Notes:

- Using a slow juicer retains more of the enzymes from the fruit and vegetables, but any type of juicer is better than none!
- If you are allergic to pears, use 1 red/golden delicious apple instead (contains medium salicylates — note that all other apples contain high salicylates so they should be avoided during the program).

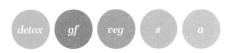

Sprout Smoothie

Serves 1 adult, preparation time 5 minutes (plus optional freezing time)

This cleansing smoothie is designed to deodorize your body and boost liver detoxification. Mung bean sprouts and parsley are highly alkalizing and rich in vitamin C, chlorophyll, vitamin K and folate. Your skin will glow!

- 1½ cups filtered water
- ¼ cup mung bean sprouts
- 2 tablespoons fresh parsley, chopped
- ½ teaspoon flaxseed oil (sa)
- 1 banana, peeled, pre-frozen and chopped (a)
- fine calcium powder (optional)

Place all the ingredients into a high-powdered blender and blend until smooth.

Variation: use rice milk instead of water and add ¼ cup raw cashews and 1 tablespoon of carob powder.

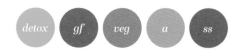
detox · gf · veg · a · ss

Body Fresh Smoothie

Serves 1 adult, preparation time 5 minutes (plus optional freezing time)

This cleansing, chlorophyll-rich smoothie is designed to deodorize your body and boost liver detoxification. Chlorella is a freshwater algae that chelates heavy metals from your body and puts a sparkle in your eyes! It contains salicylates so it's not suitable for extra sensitive people, or during the FID Program.

- 1½ cups Healthy Skin Juice (p. 187) or organic soy milk/rice milk
- 1 teaspoon pure chlorella powder (ss) (no flavouring; check ingredients)
- Skin Friend AM (optional)
- 1 small banana (a), chopped and pre-frozen (or fresh)

Place all ingredients into a high-powdered blender and blend until smooth.

Notes:
- If you find the taste of chlorella too strong, use pure barley grass powder instead. Do not use wheatgrass, spirulina or other types of green detox powders as they are very rich in salicylates, which may worsen your skin rash.
- Chlorella and barley grass often come with hidden 'natural' flavourings, fruit extracts and other additives that can worsen your skin rash, so check the ingredients and purchase 100 per cent pure powders. Note that barley grass may contain traces of gluten.
- If you are sensitive to chlorella, try the Sprout Smoothie instead (p. 187).

Dips and dressings

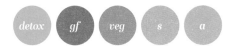

Cashew Nut Butter

Makes 1 cup, preparation time 5 minutes (plus 4+ hours soaking time)

Cashews are a rich source of zinc, manganese and copper, which assists in the production of collagen and improves your skin's ability to repair. Soak overnight to activate the nuts so their nutrients are easier to absorb.

- 1 cup raw cashews
- ½ teaspoon quality fine sea salt (or to taste)
- 1½ tablespoons Parsley Oil (p. 134) or rice bran oil
- 1 teaspoon flaxseed oil (sa)
- 3 tablespoons filtered water
- 3 g (3 scoops) fine calcium powder (optional)

Place the cashews in a sealed container and add enough water to cover them. Leave the cashews to soak for about 4 hours (or overnight), then drain and rinse the nuts to remove any residue.

Combine all the ingredients in a high-powered blender or food processor and blend until smooth. Add extra water if necessary. Store in a sealed container in the refrigerator for about a week.

Notes:
- Make this dairy-free spread calcium enriched and acid–alkaline balanced by adding fine calcium powder. For more details read the calcium information in Chapter 7.
- This cashew nut butter can be used to add flavour to soups, stews and stir fries, or used as a tasty addition to sandwiches, crackers and waffles.

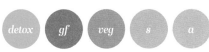

Parsley Pesto

Makes 2 small jars, preparation time 10 minutes

This protein-rich alkalizing spread is perfect for special occasions. The presence of essential fatty acids, flaxseed oil, cashews and rice bran oil makes this a powerful skin hydrating dish. Spread this dip onto plain crackers or use with vegie sticks, sourdough toast and sandwiches, or add it to pasta for a quick meal. Note: large amounts of parsley contain salicylates so eat only in moderation (if you can!).

- 1 small bunch fresh parsley
- ⅓ cup Parsley Oil (p. 134) or rice bran oil
- 2 teaspoons flaxseed oil (sa)
- 1½ cups raw cashews (preferably soaked for 4+ hours)
- 2–3 tablespoons filtered water
- 1 teaspoon freshly minced garlic, or to taste
- ½ teaspoon quality fine sea salt, or to taste

Cut half the stems off the parsley, wash the leaves in a bowl of water and shake off any excess water before placing them into a food processor. Add all the remaining ingredients and blend well. Note: do not use a high-powered blender as it will look more like avocado than pesto!

Breakfast

The following eczema-friendly breakfasts contain specially selected skin-repairing ingredients which are both nutritious and free from high levels of salicylates and other chemicals.

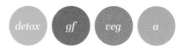

Banana Buckwheat Pancakes

Makes 8–10 pancakes, preparation time 5 minutes, cooking time 15 minutes

Bananas are a rich source of potassium, magnesium and histamine-lowering nutrients such as vitamin C. Buckwheat is a fruit seed which resembles grain and it's rich in anti-inflammatory quercetin and manganese for healthy skin. Omit the cashews if needed.

- ½ cup buckwheat flour
- 1 cup rice flour (or brown rice flour)
- 2 teaspoons baking powder (gluten-free)
- ¾ cup raw cashews (preferably soaked for 4+ hours)
- 1½–2 cups rice milk (or oat milk or gluten-free soy milk)
- 2 small–medium bananas, peeled (one sliced for decorating)
- 1 tablespoon real maple syrup (plus extra, to serve)
- rice bran oil, to oil the pan

Toppings:
Choose from: 1 large pear, peeled (t), fresh papaya, banana, Papaya Nice Cream (p. 216), Banana Nice Cream (p. 216), Cashew Nut Butter (p. 189) or Pink Pear Jam (p. 137)

Place the buckwheat flour, rice flour and baking powder into a food processor and briefly mix. Then add the soaked cashews, milk, 1 chopped banana and maple syrup and blend until smooth.

Oil a small frying pan and heat to medium–high. Using a measuring cup (¼ cup is ideal), pour in a thin layer of batter. Then, while the batter is still runny, decorate the pancake with sliced banana. Cook lightly on each side, turning when the mixture begins to bubble on top or brown underneath. Repeat the process for each pancake.

Serve with toppings of your choice.

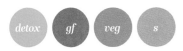

Sweet Potato Stack

Serves 1, preparation time 10 minutes, cooking time 30 minutes

Sweet potatoes are rich in vitamin C, B vitamins, manganese, and beta-carotene which is boosted with the addition of a little oil during cooking. Shallots (spring onions, scallions) are alkalizing, low in salicylates and help to prevent inflammation. Note they have a straight green stem, no rounded bulb, so don't confuse them with the bulb varieties, which are rich in salicylates. Refer to 'Specialty ingredients' photo on p. 51 to see what they look like.

- 1 small–medium sweet potato, peeled and halved lengthways (s)
- Parsley Oil, for coating (p. 134)
- quality sea salt, to taste
- ½ cup plain tofu (or black/haricot beans or free-range/organic chicken — see note)
- dried chives, to taste
- ¼ cup spring onions (shallots, scallions), finely sliced

Optional:
- 1–2 tablespoons chickpea (besan, gram) flour (if cooking chicken)
- ¼ cup fresh mung bean sprouts
- fresh chives, to serve

Preheat the oven to 200°C (400°F) and line a shallow baking tray with baking paper. Place the sweet potato on the baking tray, coat it in a little oil and sprinkle with sea salt. Roast the sweet potato for 30–40 minutes or until soft. Remove from the oven and drain on paper towels to remove any excess oil (or blot with paper towels).

Meanwhile, chop the tofu (or chicken) into bite-sized pieces and coat the tofu in a sprinkling of sea salt and chives (if using chicken, also use chickpea flour). Heat a small frying pan with a little oil on medium heat, and cook the protein until golden on each side (see notes for chicken). Remove from the heat and drain on paper towels.

Arrange the sweet potato and protein on a plate and top it with shallots, sprouts and chives.

Note: ensure the chicken is thoroughly cooked and not raw inside. For oil-free cooking, steam the seasoned tofu/chicken separately, until cooked.

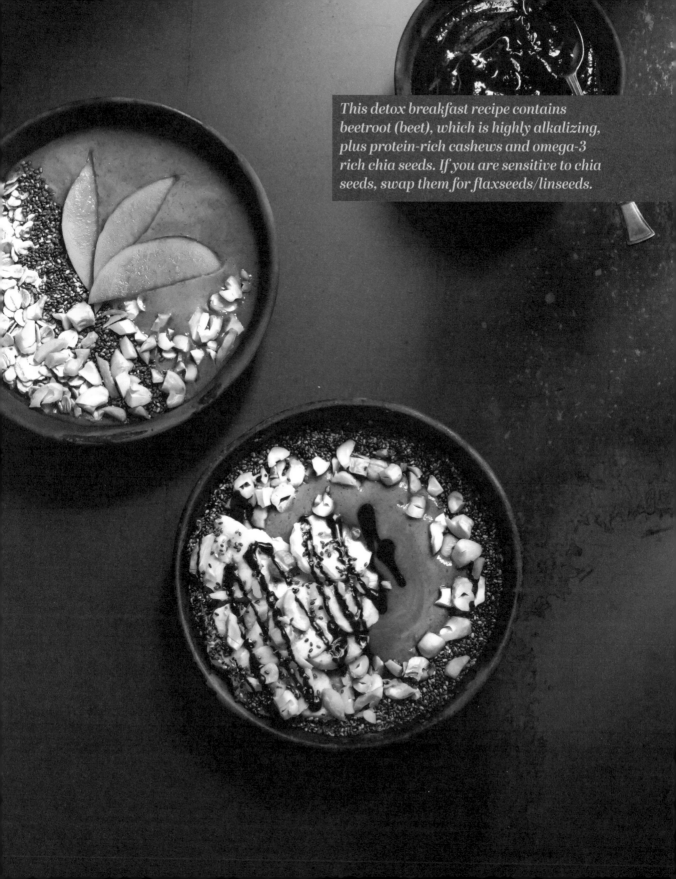

This detox breakfast recipe contains beetroot (beet), which is highly alkalizing, plus protein-rich cashews and omega-3 rich chia seeds. If you are sensitive to chia seeds, swap them for flaxseeds/linseeds.

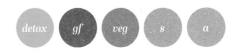

Banana Beet Smoothie Bowl

Serves 1, preparation time 5 minutes (plus overnight freezing time)

- 1 banana (a)
- ¼ cup soaked raw cashews (soaked for 4+ hours)
- ½ cup Cashew Nut Milk (p. 184) or rice milk
- 1 tablespoon grated fresh beetroot (beet), peeled (s)

Optional:
- 2 slices of papaya/pawpaw (can be pre-frozen)
- Skin Friend AM
- ½ teaspoon flaxseed oil (sa)

Toppings:
- 1 teaspoon chia seeds (sa)
- banana, pawpaw or papaya slices (a)
- raw cashews, chopped (if not allergic to nuts)

To freeze the banana, peel it first, slice into bite-sized pieces, then store in a freezer bag or sealed container.

Place all of the ingredients, except the toppings, into a high-powered blender and blend on high until smooth. Serve in a bowl and top with chia seeds, fruit and chopped cashews.

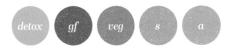

Raw Omega Muesli

Makes 5–6 servings, preparation time 7 minutes

Muesli, also known as granola, typically contains itch-promoting ingredients such as dried fruits and honey, but this version is low in natural chemicals and gluten-free if using gluten-free oats. Quinoa flakes are flattened quinoa and a good source of manganese, copper, zinc and magnesium.

- 2½ cups rolled oats (gluten-free if possible)
- 1½ cups quinoa flakes or plain puffed brown rice
- ¼ cup whole flaxseeds/linseeds
- ½ cup raw cashews, chopped in half (optional — see note)

Place the ingredients in a large sealable container and mix well. Serve with milk of choice (refer to the Eczema Detox Program shopping list on p. 92–3) and add eczema-friendly sweetener if desired.

Note: some people are sensitive to cashews and they don't realize it, so test cashews before using this ingredient (see p. 84 for test information).

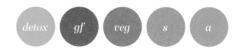

Protein Smoothie Bowl

Serves 1, preparation time 5 minutes (plus overnight freezing time)

- 1 medium banana (a)
- 1–2 tablespoons pea/rice protein powder (pure, no flavouring or fruit)
- ½ cup Cashew Nut Milk (p. 184) or rice milk or oat milk
- 1 teaspoon carob powder
- ½ teaspoon flaxseed oil (sa)

Optional:
- 2 slices papaya/pawpaw (can be pre-frozen) (a)
- real maple syrup (if extra sweetness needed)
- Skin Friend AM

Optional toppings:
- banana slices (a)
- 1 teaspoon chopped raw cashews
- chia seeds or flaxseeds/linseeds (sa)

To freeze the banana, peel it first, slice it into bite-sized pieces, then store in a freezer bag or sealed container.

Place all the ingredients, except the toppings, into a high-powered blender and blend on high until smooth. Serve in a bowl and top with banana, chopped cashews and chia seeds or flaxseeds.

Note: if you are sensitive to glutamates or MSG, you might not be able to consume protein powders as they naturally contain glutamic acid, a type of glutamate. You can test protein powder in the FID Program (see p. 84 for details).

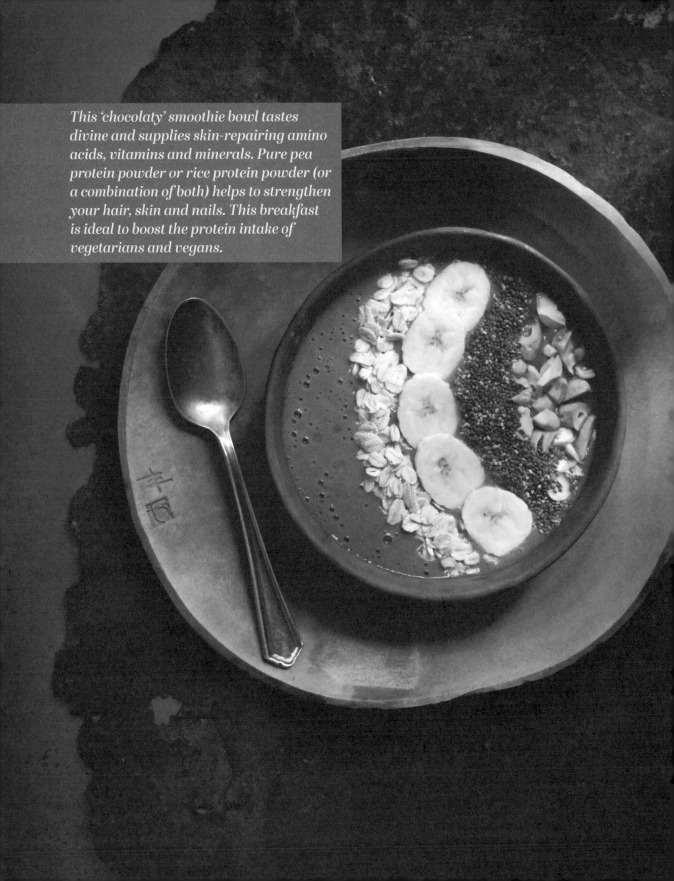

This 'chocolaty' smoothie bowl tastes divine and supplies skin-repairing amino acids, vitamins and minerals. Pure pea protein powder or rice protein powder (or a combination of both) helps to strengthen your hair, skin and nails. This breakfast is ideal to boost the protein intake of vegetarians and vegans.

Lunch and dinner

When you have skin problems it's important to eat fibre-rich foods packed with antioxidants, vitamins and minerals to boost the health of your liver and digestive system. The following nutritious recipes are designed to supply liver-detoxifying and digestive system-supporting nutrients.

There are sixteen additional FID lunch and dinner recipes to choose from, beginning on p. 152, that are also suitable for those following the Eczema Detox Program.

You can also create your own meals using the ingredients from the Eczema Detox shopping list on pp. 92–3. Feel free to cook tofu, beans, lean lamb, lean beef, skinless chicken, veal or fresh fish using the following seasonings which are low in food chemicals (do not use other seasonings):

garlic

garlic powder

chives (fresh and dried)

parsley (fresh and dried)

quality sea salt (no additives)

Celtic sea salt

Himalayan salt

iodised sea salt (not table salt)

chickpea (besan, gram) flour

rice flour (brown rice flour)

spelt flour

Pumpkin and Snow Pea (mangetout) Bowl

Serves 1–2, preparation time 10 minutes, cooking time 7 minutes

This antioxidant-rich vegetable dish is acid–alkaline balanced and makes a great grain-free breakfast or lunch. Top it with Caramelized Leek Sauce (p. 130), if desired.

- 1 cup pumpkin (winter squash), skin removed, sliced (s)
- 1 cup snow peas (mangetout), strings removed (s)
- ½ cup finely sliced red cabbage
- ½ cup plain tofu (or free-range/organic chicken, or cooked black/haricot beans)
- quality sea salt, to taste
- garlic powder, to taste
- Parsley Oil (p. 134) (optional, if cooking chicken)
- dried or fresh chives, to serve

You can roast or steam the pumpkin. Steaming method: place the pumpkin in a steaming basket. Add 3 cm (1½ in) of boiling water to a saucepan, place the steaming basket on top, and cover with a lid. Steam the pumpkin for 5 minutes, then add the snow peas and cabbage and steam for an additional 2 minutes, leaving the vegetables with a bit of crunch as they will continue to cook after removed from the heat.

Roasting method: preheat the oven to 180°C (350°F). Coat the pumpkin in 1–2 teaspoons of Parsley Oil (p. 134), then line a baking tray with baking paper. Place the pumpkin on the tray, then place in the oven and roast for 25 minutes or until soft.

Meanwhile, chop the tofu (or chicken) into bite-sized pieces and coat them in a little sea salt and garlic powder. You can steam the tofu/chicken separately to the vegetables, or alternatively place a small frying pan over medium heat and add a little oil, if using, then cook the protein until brown on each side (up to 2 minutes each side, though if using chicken ensure it is cooked through). Remove from the heat and drain on paper towels.

Before serving, top the protein with the vegetables and chives and season with sea salt.

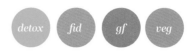

Gluten-free Besan Pastry

Makes enough for 1 large pie, preparation time 20 minutes, cooking time 30 minutes

- 1½ cups chickpea (besan, gram) flour, plus extra to flour a chopping board
- 1 teaspoon quality sea salt
- ¼ cup rice bran oil (brown rice oil)
- ¼ cup chilled filtered water (more if necessary)

Fillings:

- Lentil Sausage Rolls filling (p. 200)
- Mashed Potato (p. 162) on top of the filling
- Salmon (ss) (refer to Salmon Besan Pie, p. 207)
- Lean lamb chunks or mince with leeks and white potato etc.

Notes:

- If you are completely covering the pie with pastry, pierce it with a fork in several places — this is important to let the steam out.
- If you are using the pastry to make Lentil Sausage Rolls (p. 200) do not blind bake.

Preheat the oven to 180°C (350°F). Using a large food processor, mix together the flour and salt. Then with the motor running, add the oil through the chute, until the mixture resembles breadcrumbs. Then add the water — enough to make the dough slightly sticky (if you need more than ¼ cup, add it 1 tablespoon at a time).

Flour a large chopping board. Roll the dough until flat and thin, to about 3 mm (⅒ in) thick, into the desired shape (e.g. two round discs for a pie base and top, or square for making Lentil Sausage Rolls).

If making a pie, place the dough into a pie dish (do not stretch it) and prick holes into the base and sides using a fork. Bake the pastry first before adding the filling (known as blind baking). Tip: cover the very top rim with a strip of foil to prevent the outer edge from burning. Then bake at 180°C (350°F) for 10–15 minutes or until it looks cooked on the base (without burning the edges). Remove the pastry from the oven, leaving the oven on.

Prepare the filling of choice. Once you have assembled the pie, you can top it with Mashed Potato or thin strips of pastry arranged in a lattice pattern. Brush the top with rice milk.

Place the pie in the oven and bake for about 20 minutes or until the pastry on the top and sides is golden and crispy and the pie contents are hot. Garnish with fresh herbs and serve with Alkaline Bomb Salad (p. 153), if desired.

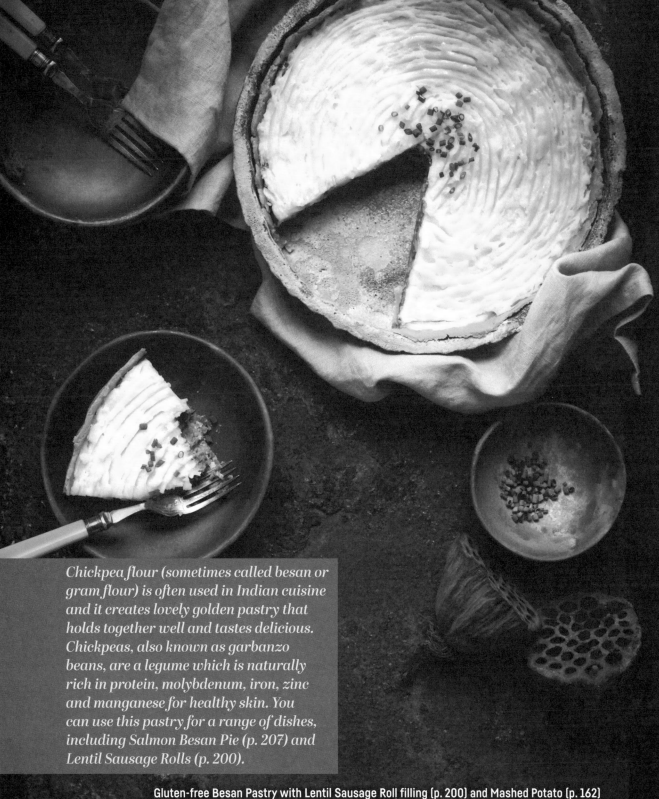

Chickpea flour (sometimes called besan or gram flour) is often used in Indian cuisine and it creates lovely golden pastry that holds together well and tastes delicious. Chickpeas, also known as garbanzo beans, are a legume which is naturally rich in protein, molybdenum, iron, zinc and manganese for healthy skin. You can use this pastry for a range of dishes, including Salmon Besan Pie (p. 207) and Lentil Sausage Rolls (p. 200).

Gluten-free Besan Pastry with Lentil Sausage Roll filling (p. 200) and Mashed Potato (p. 162)

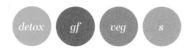

Lentil Sausage Rolls (or pie filling)

Makes 1 pie or 12 small sausage rolls, preparation time 20 minutes (plus 30 minutes to make pastry), cooking time 25 minutes

- 1 batch Gluten-free Besan Pastry (p. 198)
- 1 small–medium leek (about 1 cup when trimmed and chopped)
- 3 teaspoons Parsley Oil (p. 134) or filtered water
- 1 large clove garlic, finely chopped
- 1 medium carrot, peeled and finely diced (see notes) (s)
- 1 x 400 g (14 oz) can brown lentils, rinsed well and drained (see notes)
- ½ teaspoon garlic powder
- ½ teaspoon quality sea salt (or to taste)
- 2 tablespoons dried or fresh chives
- chia seeds, to sprinkle on top (optional)

Notes:
- If you are on the FID Program and in the first two weeks, omit the chia seeds and carrot, and use celery instead of the carrot (about ½ cup finely diced).
- If you are not using canned lentils, you will need to use 2 portions of Egg Replacer (p. 211) or two eggs (if you have tested eggs during the FID Program and found you are not sensitive to them).

Make the pastry but do not blind bake. Roll the pastry into two square sheets about 25 x 25 cm (10 x 10 in), and about 2 or 3 mm (⅒ in) thick (thinner is better) – you can roll it between two sheets of plastic wrap or on a large chopping board or clean surface. Then cover the pastry with plastic wrap and refrigerate.

Preheat the oven to 220°C (430°F) and line a baking tray with baking paper. Remove the top and bottom of the leek, then cut a slit down the middle and wash the leek (white/pale green part), removing any dirt within the layers. Finely chop the leek.

Heat a non-stick frying pan and lightly fry the leek, with a little oil or water, garlic and carrot (or celery), until the leeks are soft. Remove from the heat and place the vegetables into a food processor. Add the lentils, garlic powder, salt and chives, and mix on medium speed until the mixture sticks together. Taste and adjust the flavour if desired, adding a little more seasoning if needed.

Cut each pastry sheet in half to make four long rolls. Spoon the mixture lengthways in a line along the centre of each pastry sheet (to resemble a sausage) and fold up the sides of the pastry and pinch to seal the top.

Place the long rolls onto the baking tray and cut into desired lengths. Brush with water and sprinkle with chia seeds if desired (see notes). Bake for about 20–25 minutes or until golden and cooked.

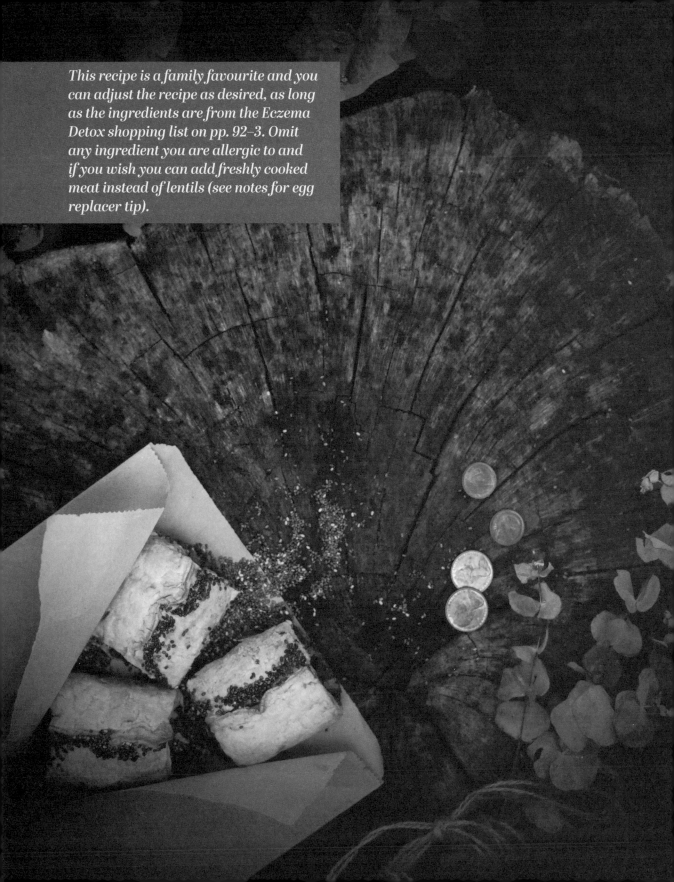

This recipe is a family favourite and you can adjust the recipe as desired, as long as the ingredients are from the Eczema Detox shopping list on pp. 92–3. Omit any ingredient you are allergic to and if you wish you can add freshly cooked meat instead of lentils (see notes for egg replacer tip).

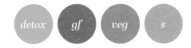

Tasty Antioxidant Coleslaw

Serves 2 as a side salad, preparation time 15 minutes

This antioxidant-rich coleslaw can be served with any type of protein including fish, lean lamb, Lentil Patties (p. 160) or Crispy Chicken Pasta (p. 176).

- 2 carrots, peeled (s)
- 1 medium beetroot (beet), peeled (s)
- 1 cup finely shredded red cabbage
- 2 tablespoons Maple Dressing (p. 135)
- 2 tablespoons Cashew Nut Butter (p. 189)

Finely grate the carrot and beetroot. Combine all the vegetables in a large bowl and set aside.

Mix the Maple Dressing with the Cashew Nut Butter to make a creamy mayonnaise. Mix the salad dressing together with vegetables just before serving.

Note: to make an FID-friendly version of this recipe use spring onions (shallots, scallions; straight stem, no rounded bulb), celery, parsley, red cabbage and Maple Dressing (p. 135).

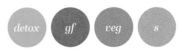

Roasted Sweet Potato Salad

Serves 1 (or 2 as a side dish), preparation time 10 minutes, cooking time 30–40 minutes

Sweet potatoes are rich in beta-carotene, which helps to protect your skin from UV sun damage, plus vitamin C, manganese, copper, vitamin B5 and vitamin B6 for skin repair and maintenance. Serve this dish with healthy protein foods such as beans, tofu, skinless chicken, fresh fish or lean lamb.

- 1 small sweet potato, halved lengthways (s)
- ½ teaspoon Parsley Oil (p. 134) or rice bran oil
- quality sea salt (fine), to taste
- Sesame-free Hummus (p. 132) or Maple Dressing (p. 135), to serve
- cos (romaine) lettuce leaves (s) (or iceberg lettuce), as desired
- handful of mung bean sprouts
- sprinkling of raw cashews, halved (optional)

Preheat the oven to 200°C (400°F). In a shallow roasting pan, coat the potato with a little oil (do not let the potato sit in oil) and sprinkle with fine sea salt. Roast for 30 minutes or until very soft on the inside.

Meanwhile, make the dip or dressing if not already made. Serve the sweet potato with salad leaves and a dollop of dip (or 1 teaspoon salad dressing). Top with sprouts and cashews.

Note: to make this dish FID-friendly, use peeled white potato instead of sweet potato and iceberg lettuce instead of cos.

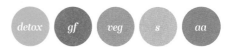

Sweet Potato Soup

Serves 6, preparation time 20 minutes, cooking time 30 minutes

Delicious and creamy, sweet potato soup is a low GI version of pumpkin soup (which is high GI). Research shows that adding about 5 grams of oil when cooking sweet potato enhances the uptake of beta-carotene, providing all your daily needs of vitamin A, plus half your recommended daily intake of vitamin C and manganese.

- 1 leek, white part only
- 3 Brussels sprouts, finely chopped
- 1–2 teaspoons Parsley Oil (p. 134) or rice bran oil
- 1.2 kg (2½ lb) sweet potatoes (the orange variety, see notes) (s)
- 2 cloves garlic, minced
- 3 cups Therapeutic Broth (p. 205) (aa), or Alkaline Vegetable Broth (p. 167) or use filtered water instead
- 4 cups filtered water
- ½ cup dried red split lentils
- ½ teaspoon quality sea salt, or to taste
- Cashew Nut Butter, p. 189 (optional)

Wash the leek and ensure you remove any dirt from the upper layers then finely chop. In a large deep saucepan, sauté the leek and Brussels sprouts in 1 teaspoon of oil for 2 minutes. Peel and chop the sweet potatoes, then add them to the saucepan along with the garlic and a splash more oil and sauté for another 5 minutes. Then add the broth and water, cover and bring to the boil.

Meanwhile, prepare the lentils by rinsing them thoroughly in a large bowl of water, then drain them and remove any discoloured ones. Add them to the saucepan, then cover and simmer for 25–30 minutes, adding another cup of water if necessary. Season with salt (add a little extra if you are using water instead of broth).

Remove the saucepan from the heat and allow the soup to cool for 5–10 minutes. Using a blender or food processor, blend the soup in batches to make it smooth. Add another ½ cup or more of water if necessary. Serve in bowls and, if desired, top with a swirl of Cashew Nut Butter.

Notes: 1.2 kg (2½ lb) is approximately four large sweet potatoes. If you want fewer salicylates use three sweet potatoes and four medium white potatoes (peel off the skin and ensure you remove all the green parts, if any).

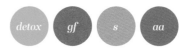
Steamed Salmon with Maple Dressing

Serves 2, preparation time 15 minutes, cooking time 30 minutes

Eat fish once or twice a week as it is one of the best foods for healthy skin, providing vitamin D, zinc, protein and omega-3. Omega-3 fatty acids are important for brain development and can reduce the risk of eczema and asthma. Spring onions (shallots, scallions), leeks and cabbage provide powerful compounds that promote liver detoxification. Read the notes below before buying the fish.

- 1 medium sweet potato, peeled and halved lengthways (s)
- 1 teaspoon Parsley Oil (p. 134) or rice bran oil
- quality sea salt, to taste
- garlic powder (optional), to taste
- Maple Dressing (p. 135)
- 1 large fresh salmon fillet, halved (or refer to fish list on p. 92)
- 1 carrot, peeled and finely julienned (see notes) (s)
- handful of snow peas (mangetout), strings removed (s)
- ½ cup finely shredded red cabbage
- 1 spring onion (shallots, scallions; straight green stem, no rounded bulb)

Preheat the oven to 200°C (400°F) and line a baking tray with baking paper. Coat the sweet potato in the oil and season with sea salt and garlic powder. Place the sweet potato on the baking tray and bake in the oven for 30 minutes or until soft and golden.

Meanwhile, make the Maple Dressing if you haven't done so already. Use ¼ cup of the dressing to coat the fish, then place the fish in a sealed container and put in the refrigerator to marinate for 10 minutes. Then using a steamer, simmer 2 cups water and place the fish into the steamer basket. Top with garlic powder. Cover and steam the fish for about 5 minutes or until just cooked through (cooking time will vary depending on the thickness of the fish). If the fish develops white clumps it means you have overcooked it. Remove from the heat, and transfer the fish to a plate and cover.

Clean the basket and then steam the carrots, snow peas and red cabbage for 2 minutes. Finely chop the spring onion and set aside. Serve the fish with the baked sweet potato, topped with sea salt and 1 teaspoon of Maple Dressing per person. Garnish with spring onions.

Notes:
- If you are following the FID Program, omit the salmon and choose smaller white fish (fresh, not frozen) such as flathead or silver dory, and omit the sweet potato, carrot and snow peas (mangetout) and have white potato and green beans instead.
- Julienned carrots are very thin strips that resemble matchsticks.

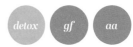

Therapeutic Broth

Makes 6–8 cups, preparation time 6 minutes, cooking time 5 hours, make 1 day before use (see notes)

- 2 large beef or lamb bones (with a little meat on them: necks, joints, marrow)
- 3.5 litres (7 pt) filtered water (at room temperature)
- 1 large chicken carcass (bones or necks etc.)
- ½ teaspoon ascorbic acid or 1 teaspoon malt vinegar (a)
- ½ large leek, white part only
- 2 spring onions (shallots, scallions; straight stem, no rounded bulb), ends trimmed and chopped
- 3 Brussels sprouts
- 2 stalks celery
- 3 cloves garlic, minced
- 1 teaspoon quality sea salt

Notes:
- This recipe contains amines.
- Wash all vegetables and choose organic meats if available.
- Do not use other types of vinegar as they contain higher amines.
- Broth will last for a week if refrigerated and can be used in soups etc.
- Store the leftover broth in clean glass jars or containers, and freeze the leftovers.
- Freeze 1 tablespoon portions into ice cube trays for use in children's meals.

Preheat the oven to 200°C (400°F). Place the beef bones in a roasting pan and roast for 30 minutes.

Remove the beef bones from the oven and add them to a large pot along with the water, chicken bones and ascorbic acid or malt vinegar. The acid helps to extract the minerals from the bones. Allow the bones to soak, without turning on the heat, to give the acid time to work, while you wash and chop the vegetables (the smaller the pieces, the more nutrients extracted). Bring the pot to the boil and add the vegetables and remaining ingredients and simmer over a low heat, covered with a lid, for 4–6 hours.

After the first hour of cooking, break apart the bones using tongs, to allow more of the minerals to be extracted. The broth will be more flavoursome if it reduces by half but if the water evaporates too much, add more water.

After 4–6 hours remove the bones from the broth (the chicken bones be soft and brittle by now). Place a strainer over a large bowl then pour the broth through the strainer, discarding the remaining bones and vegetables when you have finished. Squeeze out as much liquid as possible as you strain the broth.

The next step is very important. Store the broth in the refrigerator overnight so the fat has time to solidify on top of the broth. The next day carefully skim off the hard layer of fat (this saturated fat is not good for your eczema so it all has to go). If your broth is thick and jelly-like it means it is rich in collagen (gelatin), which is full of glycine and other nutrients required for healthy skin.

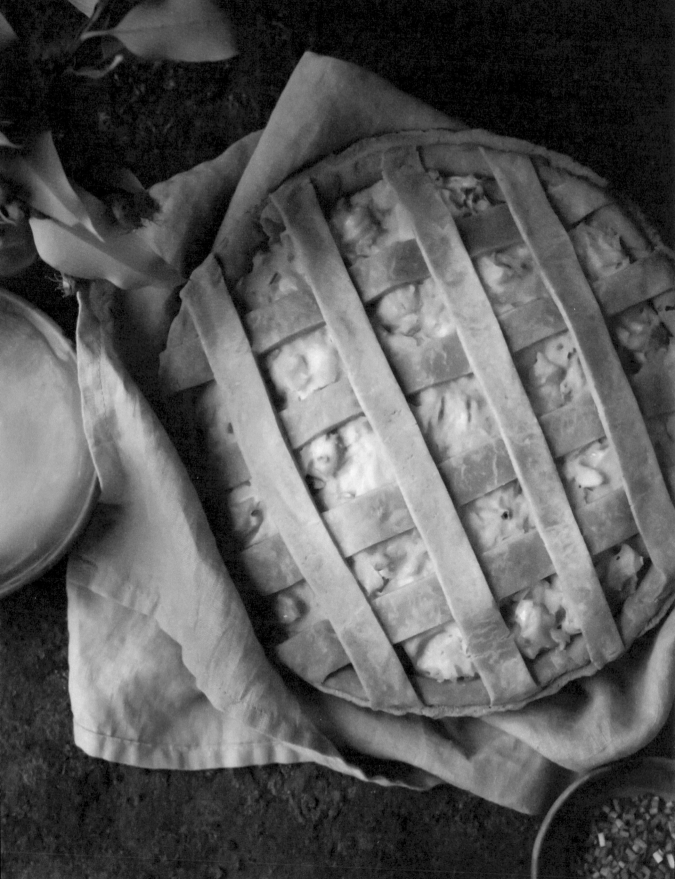

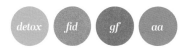

Salmon Besan Pie

Makes 1 large pie, preparation time 30 minutes, cooking time 35 minutes

Salmon is a beautiful fish that's rich in protein for healthy hair and nails, and skin-moisturizing omega-3 fatty acids to calm skin inflammation. Garnish this pie with fresh chives and serve with Tasty Antioxidant Coleslaw (p. 202), if desired. If you are following the FID Program, use fresh white fish instead of salmon and avoid nuts.

- Gluten-free Besan Pastry base (p. 198)
- 4 large white potatoes, peeled
- ½–¾ cup Cashew Nut Milk (p. 184) or rice milk or organic soy milk
- 2 medium-sized leeks, tops cut off
- 2 teaspoons Parsley Oil (p. 134) or rice bran oil
- 2 cloves fresh garlic, minced
- 1 teaspoon garlic powder
- 1 teaspoon quality sea salt
- 1 x 250–300 g (9–10½ oz) skinless salmon fillet (deboned) (aa)
- 1 tablespoon finely chopped chives
- 1 tablespoon finely chopped parsley
- 1 tablespoon finely chopped spring onions (shallots, scallions: thin green stems, no bulb)

Preheat the oven to 180°C (350°F). Prepare the pastry base and blind bake it as per the instruction on p. 198. Lattice pastry strips, used to decorate the top of the pie, can be made prior so the pie can be topped quickly and placed in oven. Make the strips about 2 cm (1 in) wide, and about 3 mm (⅒ in) thick (do not blind bake the strips).

Cube the potatoes and boil until soft, then mash with Cashew Nut Milk until slightly chunky.

Wash the leeks and ensure there is no dirt in the layers and slice finely. Place a frying pan over a medium heat and add the oil. Add the leeks and caramelize, adding a little more oil or water if needed, then add the garlic during the last minute of cooking. Add the potato mixture to the leeks and garlic, then stir in the garlic powder and salt.

Dice the salmon into small 1 cm (½ in) cubes. Stir the salmon pieces, chives, parsley and spring onions through the potato mixture. Then place into the pie dish and top with lattice pastry.

Place the pie in oven and bake for about 20 minutes or until the pastry on top is golden and crispy and the pie contents are hot.

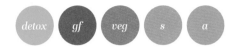

Papaya Rice Paper Rolls

Makes about 20 rolls, preparation time 40 minutes

- 300 g (10½ oz) plain tofu or skinless free-range chicken, thinly sliced
- freshly minced garlic or dried garlic powder, to taste
- quality sea salt, to taste
- packet round rice paper (20 sheets or 250 g/9 oz)
- ½ ripe papaya (a), skin and seeds discarded, thinly sliced
- 3 handfuls finely shredded cos (romaine) (s) or iceberg lettuce
- 2 medium carrots, grated (s)
- mung bean sprouts (freshest only), washed thoroughly

Mix the tofu or chicken with a sprinkling of garlic and salt and place in a steamer basket. Steam for 5 minutes or until thoroughly cooked (if using chicken, ensure it is cooked through). Remove from the heat and allow to partially cool.

Wet a clean tea towel, wring out the excess water and place flat on the kitchen bench. Soften the rice paper, one at a time, in a large bowl of very warm water, soaking each sheet for 10–20 seconds. Remove the rice paper before it gets too soft and place flat on the damp tea towel. Arrange the tofu (or chicken) papaya, lettuce, carrot and sprouts in a row, on the rice paper near the end closest to you, then roll it up, tucking the ends in about halfway so they look like cylinders (also refer to the rice paper packaging for instructions).

Note: refer to the photo for additional eczema-friendly fillings, including parsley, grated beetroot (beets; s) and red cabbage, and for dipping sauces use Maple Dressing (p. 135) or Parsley Pesto (p. 189).

This recipe is delicious and delicate and perfectly acid–alkaline balanced thanks to the mung bean sprouts, which are highly alkalizing.

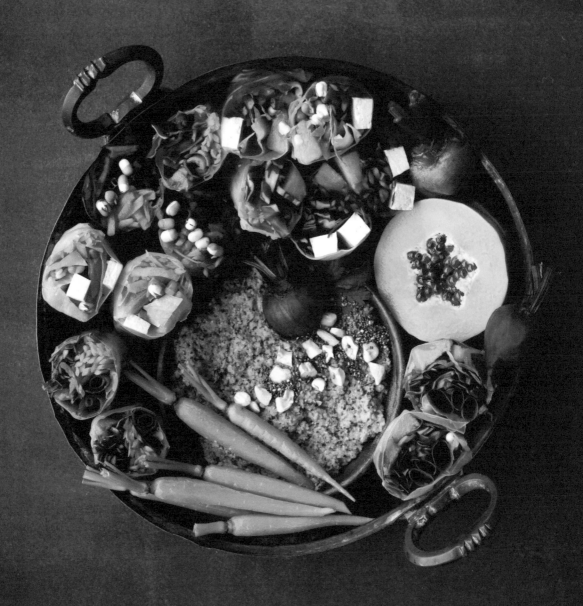

Simple San Choy Bau

Serves 2–4 children, preparation time 10 minutes, cooking time 12 minutes

This simple children's version of the classic Chinese favourite will win over even the fussiest child. Instead of organic lamb mince you can use chicken or turkey mince, tofu or black (haricot) beans. If you are following the FID Program, omit the carrot and replace it with celery or shredded iceberg lettuce.

- ½ cup white rice (not jasmine or basmati)
- 1 teaspoon Parsley Oil (p. 134)
- 250 g (9 oz) preservative-free organic lamb mince
- 1 tablespoon dried or fresh parsley
- quality sea salt, to taste
- 4–6 medium, whole iceberg lettuce leaves, to serve
- 1 carrot, peeled and grated (s)
- Maple Dressing (optional, p. 135), to serve

Cook the rice in a saucepan of boiling water according to the packet instructions (about 10 minutes). Drain and set aside to cool.

Place a frying pan over high heat and add the oil. Add the mince and break it apart to prevent lumps. Cook, stirring occasionally, until the mince has separated and browned. Add the parsley and salt and reduce the heat to low, then continue cooking until the meat is cooked through and no longer pink.

Ensure the rice is not hot as it will wilt the lettuce leaves. Place the lettuce leaves on plates and fill with the rice, mince and grated carrot. Drizzle a teaspoon of Maple Dressing onto each lettuce cup and serve.

Snacks and lunchbox

Choose from the following snacks and lunchbox items and remember to include at least five serves of alkalizing vegetables. Choose from additional snacks from the FID Program, including Potato and Leek Waffles (p. 147) and Oat Waffles (p. 145).

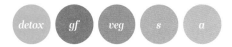

Egg Replacer

Equivalent to 1 egg, preparation time 15 minutes

Use ground flaxseeds/linseeds to replace eggs in the recipes. Flaxseeds are anti-inflammatory and rich in omega-3 and mucilage to soothe your intestinal tract and promote healing. Note that flaxseeds contain medium salicylates and amines, so avoid using them if you are highly sensitive to these compounds. Double the recipe if replacing two eggs.

- 1 tablespoon whole flaxseeds/linseeds (sa)
- 2 tablespoons filtered water

Grind the flaxseeds to a fine powder using a high-powered blender or seed/coffee grinder. Mix the powder with the filtered water in a small bowl and refrigerate for 10 minutes to thicken.

Banana Bread

Makes 1 loaf, preparation time 20 minutes, cooking time 50 minutes

This delicious banana bread is amazing served freshly toasted. It can also be made with regular gluten-free flour (check ingredients are low salicylates). Ensure the bananas are ripe enough to mash. If you are sensitive to eggs or flaxseeds/linseeds omit them, as banana also acts as a binder.

- 2 free-range/organic eggs, whisked, or 2 x Egg Replacer (p. 211) (optional)
- 1 cup brown rice flour
- ½ cup quinoa flour
- pinch of quality sea salt
- 3 teaspoons baking powder (gluten-free)
- 3 very ripe small–medium bananas, mashed (approx. 1½ cups) (a)
- ½ cup real maple syrup or rice malt syrup (brown rice syrup)
- 2 tablespoons brown rice oil (rice bran oil)
- 1 teaspoon real vanilla essence (optional)

Make the Egg Replacer if using and set aside in the refrigerator. Preheat the oven to 170°C (325°F).

Sift into a large bowl the two flours, salt and baking powder, then mix. In another large bowl, mash the bananas with a fork or potato masher, then stir in the maple syrup, Egg Replacer or egg, oil and vanilla essence and mix together. Add the wet mixture to the dry ingredients and fold together, being careful not to over-mix.

Line a rectangular loaf tin (approx. 13 x 24 cm/ 5 x 9½ in) with baking paper. Pour in the mixture and bake for 40–50 minutes or until set and golden on top. It may seem a little undercooked when it comes out but it will firm slightly.

To serve: this banana bread needs to be toasted just before serving so cut thick slices (about 2 cm/1 in thick) and toast in a toaster or lightly fry in a pan until golden on each side. Serve on its own or with Pink Pear Jam (p. 137), Cashew Nut Butter (p. 189) or one of the Nice Cream recipes on p. 216.

Recipe from Katie Layland.

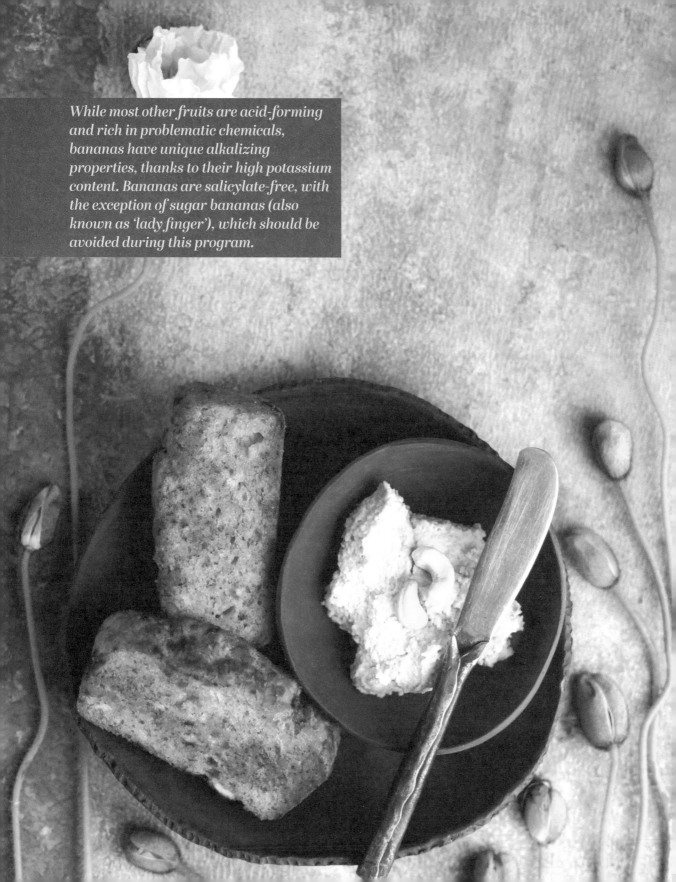

While most other fruits are acid-forming and rich in problematic chemicals, bananas have unique alkalizing properties, thanks to their high potassium content. Bananas are salicylate-free, with the exception of sugar bananas (also known as 'lady finger'), which should be avoided during this program.

Desserts

The following desserts are healthy, nutritious and rich in antioxidants.

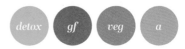

Caramelized Bananas

Serves 1, preparation time 2 minutes, cooking time 4 minutes

- 1 medium banana, peeled (a)
- real maple syrup (or rice malt syrup/brown rice syrup)

Cut the banana in half and then slice lengthwise. Add a couple of teaspoons of syrup to a non-stick frying pan and spread to coat. Place on a medium heat and add the sliced bananas. Reduce the heat to medium–low, cook for 2–3 minutes until golden, and flip. Cook for 1 more minute, reduce the heat to low and allow to cook until very soft.

Eat for dessert, or serve on top of oatmeal.
Recipe by Charlie Rioux.

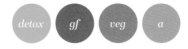

Banana Carob Icy Poles

Serves 5, preparation time 5 minutes (plus overnight freezing time)

- 2–3 large ripe bananas, mashed (a)
- 2 tablespoons carob powder
- 2 teaspoons real maple syrup (optional)
- ¼ cup organic rice milk (or organic soy milk)
- 3 g (3 scoops) fine calcium powder (optional)

Using a wooden spoon, mix all the ingredients together in a large bowl, or for smooth icy poles use a food processor. Add an extra splash of rice milk if needed, until you achieve the desired consistency. Freeze in ice block moulds and serve once hard (let them set overnight).

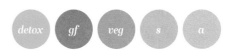
Carob Chia Pudding

Serves 4, preparation time 10 minutes (plus overnight setting time)

Carob is a healthy, caffeine-free alternative to chocolate. It is free of amines and salicylates, and rich in an antioxidant tannin called gallic acid, which has impressive anti-allergic properties. Chia seeds are a great source of anti-inflammatory omega-3, dietary fibre and mucilage which becomes jelly-like in liquids, making them perfect for setting puddings. If you are following the FID Program, use sago instead of chia seeds — you will need to cook sago so read the notes for instructions.

- 1½ cups Cashew Nut Milk (p. 184) (or organic soy milk or rice milk)
- ¼ cup carob powder
- 3–4 tablespoons real maple syrup (or rice malt syrup)
- 3 g (3 scoops) fine calcium powder (optional, see notes)
- ⅓ cup chia seeds (sa) (or sago; see notes)

Place the milk, carob, syrup and calcium powder into a food processor or blender and blend until smooth. Taste and adjust the sweetness if necessary. Stir in the chia seeds (they are lovely kept whole but if you prefer you can blend these as well). Place in decorative jars or bowls, cover and refrigerate until set.

Notes:

- Sago pudding recipe for people on the FID Program: simmer the sago and milk in a saucepan on low heat for 15 minutes, covered, or until the sago becomes translucent. In a cup, mix the carob powder with 1 tablespoon of boiling water. Then add the carob, syrup and calcium (and extra liquid if needed) to the sago and mix. Refrigerate until set.
- Fine calcium powder can be added for acid–alkaline balance whenever sweetener is used (see 'Useful resources', p. 220).
- Do not use chocolate, cocoa or cacao as they are rich in caffeine and fats, which can worsen skin rashes and increase skin dryness and irritation.
- Drink a full glass of filtered water when eating chia seeds as they soak up a lot of liquid.

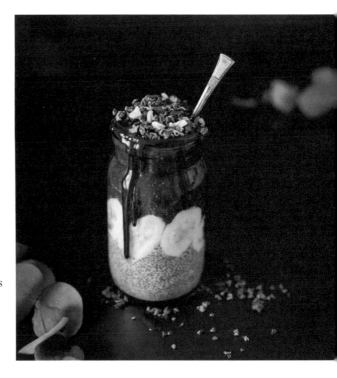

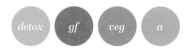

Papaya Nice Cream

Serves 2, preparation time 5 minutes (plus overnight freezing time)

Half a medium papaya provides 100 per cent of your body's daily vitamin C needs, plus folate, beta-carotene, magnesium and vitamin B5 for clear skin. Papaya is a digestive aid that promotes healthy gut flora. This Nice Cream has a sublime, smooth consistency of whipped sorbet.

- 1 medium-sized papaya (skin removed, chopped and pre-frozen overnight) (a)
- 1 tablespoon pure maple syrup or rice malt syrup (brown rice syrup) (optional)
- 1 tablespoon rice milk or Cashew Nut Milk (p. 184)

Place the frozen papaya pieces into a food processor. Add the syrup and milk and blend on medium speed. Scrape the sides down and blend again. You should not need to add more milk if blending for a couple of minutes on medium speed (not high), but add a tablespoon extra if needed. The consistencey should be of soft serve — if you would like it to be firm, place it in the freezer for an hour or more. Serve immediately. Leftovers can be placed into ice block moulds and stored in the freezer for 2–3 days.

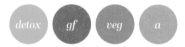

Banana Nice Cream

Serves 2, preparation time 5 minutes (plus overnight freezing time)

- 2 large ripe bananas (peeled, chopped and pre-frozen overnight) (a)
- 1 tablespoon rice milk or Cashew Nut Milk (p. 184)
- 1 tablespoon pure maple syrup or rice malt syrup (optional)

Place the frozen bananas into a food processor. Add the milk and maple syrup and blend on medium speed. Scrape the sides down and blend again. You should not need to add more milk if blending for a couple of minutes on medium speed (not high), but add a tablespoon extra if needed. Do not add too much liquid or it will become runny (if this occurs, place the Nice Cream into the freezer for about 20 minutes). The consistency should be of soft serve — if you would like it to be firm, place it in the freezer for an hour or more. Serve immediately. Leftovers can be placed into ice block moulds and stored in the freezer for 1–2 days.

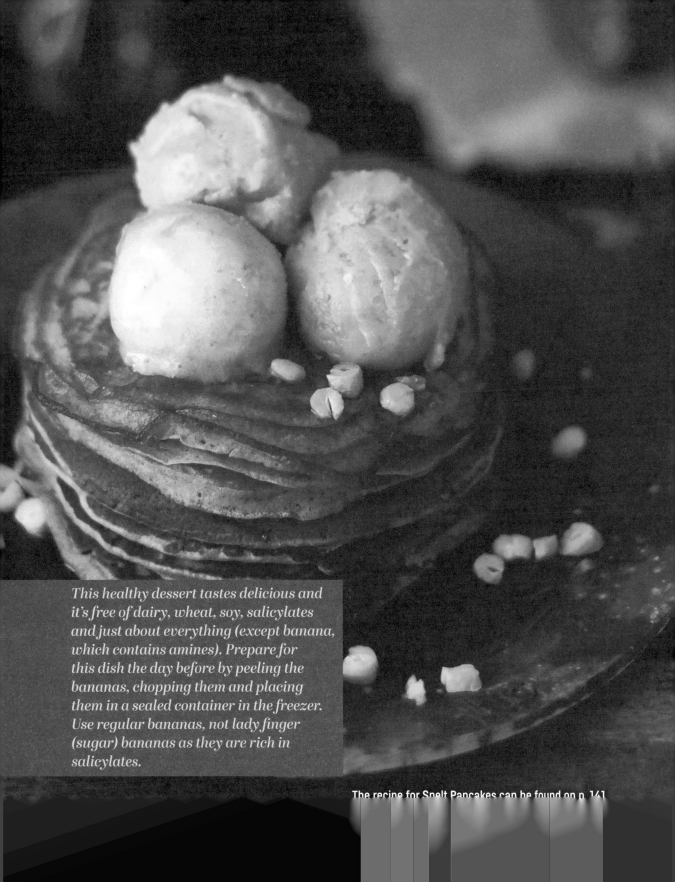

This healthy dessert tastes delicious and it's free of dairy, wheat, soy, salicylates and just about everything (except banana, which contains amines). Prepare for this dish the day before by peeling the bananas, chopping them and placing them in a sealed container in the freezer. Use regular bananas, not lady finger (sugar) bananas as they are rich in salicylates.

The recipe for Spelt Pancakes can be found on p. 141

Chapter 15
Recipe and test foods: salicylate test

Following is a 'high-salicylate' test recipe you can use to test for salicylate sensitivity (during weeks 3–4 of the FID Program), plus a list of testing foods you can try. If you know you are highly sensitive to salicylate do not test salicylates.

High-salicylate test foods

Here are the high-salicylate foods that are suitable for salicylate testing as they do not contain amines or MSG.

High-salicylate fruits	High-salicylate vegetables	High-salicylate herbs and spices
Apples, apricot, blueberries, cherries, rockmelon (cantaloupe), guava, lychee, melons, nectarine, pomegranate, watermelon	Alfalfa sprouts, artichoke, capsicum (bell pepper), chicory, cucumber, endive, onions, water chestnuts, watercress, zucchini (courgette)	Bay leaf, coriander (cilantro), mint, rosemary (most herbs); aniseed, caraway, cardamom, cinnamon, cloves, five spice, ginger, mace, nutmeg, paprika, pepper, turmeric

How to choose and de-seed a pomegranate

When shopping for a pomegranate, choose a nice heavy one that has firm, unwrinkled skin with no decaying or softened patches. The easy way to de-seed a pomegranate involves submerging it in water — this prevents everything from staining red and the seeds sink to the bottom, while the white pith floats to the top.

1. Place the pomegranate in a bowl of water. Using a sharp knife, cut the top off the pomegranate. You can do this in one long shallow cut about 0.5 cm (⅕ in) deep, following the outer ridge at the top. Or you can do this in four cuts, like a square lid.
2. Lift the lid off the pomegranate and remove any seeds attached to the lid and place them in the water.
3. Note the wedge formations inside the pomegranate caused by the white pith. Shallow cut the skin of the pomegranate following the natural wedge lines — there will be about five wedges.
4. Break the wedges apart and gently remove the seeds while in the water.
5. Scoop out the floating pith and discard any damaged, discoloured or whitish seeds, then strain the remaining seeds and drain well.

Quinoa and Pomegranate Salad

Serves 2 (or 4 as a side dish), preparation time 20 minutes, cooking time 15 minutes

This antioxidant-rich salad is a classic dinner party dish, with a delicate balance of flavours. Ingredients with high levels of salicylates are denoted with (SS). You can add Maple Dressing (p. 135) to this salad.

- 1 cup red or white quinoa, rinsed
- 1 large pomegranate (ss), seeds removed (see p. 218)
- quality sea salt, to taste
- 2 teaspoons extra virgin olive oil (ss) or Parsley Oil (p. 134)
- ½ cup raw cashews, chopped
- 1 cup finely chopped mint leaves (ss)

Place the quinoa into a saucepan with 2½ cups of water, cover and bring to the boil. Then simmer on low heat for approximately 12–15 minutes or until the grains have softened.

Meanwhile, remove the seeds from the pomegranate. You will need 1 cup pomegranate seeds.

Drain the quinoa and allow to cool. Place in a serving bowl, sprinkle on the oil and mix. Add the pomegranate seeds, cashews and mint and lightly toss.

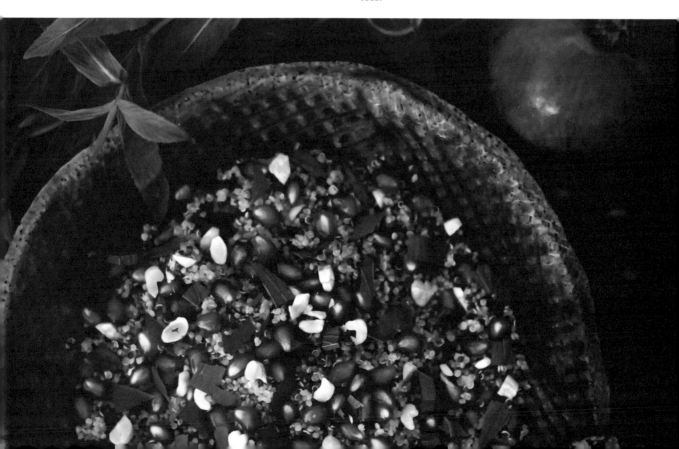

The last word ...

I hope this book helps to clear the confusion and empower you to heal your skin inflammation from the inside out so you can live a happy, healthy (and normal!) life.

Useful resources

Eczema Life Clinic, Sydney, Australia

Karen Fischer's clinic
By appointment only
support@eczemalife.com
www.eczemalife.com

Vitamin and mineral supplements

Skin Friend AM
Contains magnesium, zinc, vitamin B6, biotin, vitamin B12 (and other B vitamins), taurine, choline, inositol, vitamin C and molybdenum etc. www.skinfriend.com

Skin Friend PM
Fine calcium powder (with magnesium and glycine) www.skinfriend.com

Other supplements
www.eczemalife.com (search 'eczema supplements' for products and links — these are updated regularly)

pH test kit

Test your acid–alkaline balance
Skin Friend pH Kit
www.skinfriend.com

Eczema information for pregnancy and breastfeeding
www.skinfriend.com (search 'pregnancy' or 'breastfeeding')

Diet diary
www.skinfriend.com (search 'diet diary')

Facebook

The Eczema Diet page
www.facebook.com/TheEczemaDiet

Eczema Diet support group
www.facebook.com/groups/
EczemaDietSupport/

Instagram
@eczema.life
@laneandspoon

Red skin syndrome/topical steroid withdrawal support group
www.itsan.org

Skincare balms and bath products for eczema
www.skinfriend.com

Associations

Eczema Association of Australasia
www.eczema.org.au

Eczema Scotland
www.eczemascotland.org

Eczema Society of Canada
https://eczemahelp.ca

European Federation of Allergy and Airways Diseases Patients Association
www.efanet.org

National Eczema Association (USA)
www.nationaleczema.org

National Eczema Society (UK)
www.eczema.org

Additional recipes

Fischer, Karen, 2012, *The Eczema Diet: Eczema-safe food to stop the itch and prevent eczema for life*, Exisle Publishing. Available at www.exislepublishing.com or www.skinfriend.com
Swain, A.R. and Loblay, R.H., 2002, *Friendly Food: The essential guide to avoiding allergies, additives and problem chemicals*, Murdoch Books, Sydney.

Sweet Salty Spicy
Charlie Rioux's blog
www.sweetsaltyspicy.net
(click on the 'dietary needs' tab, then click on 'The Eczema Diet')

Eczema Life
Karen Fischer's blog
www.eczemalife.com

Feeding fussy children

Fischer, Karen, 2010, *Healthy Family, Happy Family: The complete guide to feeding your family*, Exisle Publishing. Available at www.exislepublishing.com

Low-salicylate toothpastes

www.eczemalife.com (search 'toothpaste' for brands)

Allergy tests

Ask your doctor for a referral for allergy testing in your area.

Specialty ingredients

The Australian Carob Co.
www.australiancarobs.com

The Source Bulk Foods (Australia)
Carob, chickpea (besan, gram) flour and other specialty flours
www.thesourcebulkfoods.com.au

Also Google for suppliers in your area.

Additional shopping lists are available via the product page at www.skinfriend.com. To download your free copy, use the code DETOX101 during checkout.

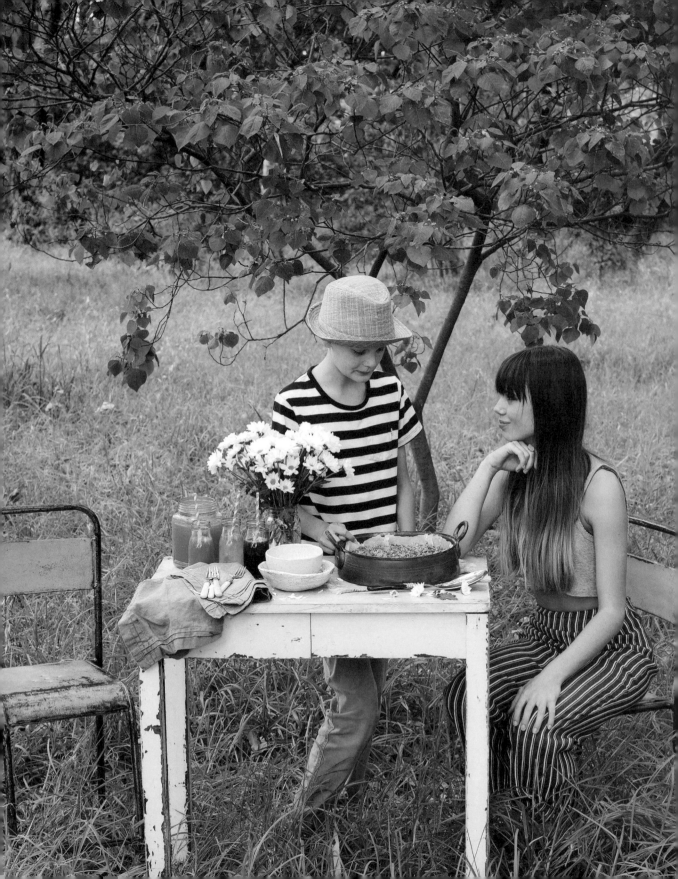

Acknowledgments

I have many people to thank for their input during the creation of *The Eczema Detox*. Firstly, my daughter Ayva, who was the initial inspiration for my eczema research. Both Ayva and Jack are wonderful (and brutally honest) recipe testers — if they didn't love the recipe it did not make it into the book. My mother is my greatest support and I can't thank her enough for her love and cooking advice, and my dad for helping me to craft some of the wooden food props which were used in the photos. It's been great getting to know you.

I wish I could have published this work ten years ago but I had much to learn. I want to personally thank my eczema patients. I could not have completed this book without working with you. The eczema sufferers who came back time and time again until we 'cracked the code' and discovered their unique food sensitivities, helped me to shape the FID Program. Clearing up eczema can be incredibly hard and disheartening so I want to thank everyone who emailed me over the years and posted social media comments letting me know their eczema cleared up. Your stories often brought tears to my eyes. I cannot name you all here but I want to say a special thank you to Charlie Rioux for sharing your eczema journey in this book and for helping others via our Facebook support group, and for your lovely recipes (the Potato and Leek Waffles are divine!). Thank you Jenny Watson, Lizzie Hunter, Georgie Broos (and Keith and Miryan), Jana and everyone who shared their success stories, and Anna for sharing your before and after photos in this book.

Thank you to our wonderful team at the Eczema Life Clinic: Sasha and Adrian Paul, Katie and Deb. I am so grateful for Katie Layland's food prep and recipes (you must try her banana bread), and for Sarah Molden's recipe testing and her mini-testing crew (hello Ava and Lily), and Deb Wiseman's recipe input (try her lovely San Choy Bau).

Selwa Anthony, thank you for believing in my writing and thanks to Benny and Gareth St John Thomas and the team at Exisle Publishing for publishing my books. The talented Tracey Gibbs made the book look beautiful, and thank you to my editors Anouska Jones and Karen Gee — I feel blessed having gluten-intolerant editors who understand health!

A heartfelt thank you to Dr Gary (Professor Gary Leong) from the Lady Cilento Children's Hospital in Queensland — thank you for your testimonials and encouragement over the years (I'm glad your cousin's eczema cleared up!).

I would also like to express my gratitude to the researchers at the RPA Hospital Allergy Unit in Sydney, especially Dr Soutter, Dr Swain and Dr Loblay, for their research on salicylates and amines (see *Friendly Food* for their work), and Sue Dengate for her research on food additives (see *Fed Up* for her work).

To you, the reader: I am humbled that you are reading this book and thank you for putting your trust in me. I hope your eczema heals swiftly. And if it does, spread the word so more people know about drug-free solutions for eczema.

Much love,
Karen

Endnotes

1. Foods that bite

1. Price, W., 2010, 'Plants bite back: The surprising, all-natural anti-nutrients and toxins in plant foods', *Sign of the Times*, retrieved from: www.sott.net
2. Loblay, R.H. and Swain, A.R., 2006, 'Food Intolerance', *Recent Advances in Clinical Nutrition*, retrieved from: www.slhd.nsw.gov.au/rpa/Allergy/research/foodintolerance_racn.pdf
3. ibid.
4. Settipane, G.A., 1990, 'History of Aspirin Intolerance,' in *Allergy and Asthma Proceedings*, vol. 11, no. 5, pp. 251–2.
5. ibid.
6. Feingold, B.F., 1975, 'Hyperkinesis and learning disabilities linked to artificial food flavors and colors', *American Journal of Nursing*, vol. 75, no. 5, pp. 797–803.
7. Loblay, R.H. and Swain, A.R., 2006, 'Food Intolerance', *Recent Advances in Clinical Nutrition*, retrieved from: www.slhd.nsw.gov.au/rpa/Allergy/research/foodintolerance_racn.pdf
8. ibid.
9. Warin, R.P. and Smith, R.J., 1976. 'Challenge test battery in chronic urticaria', *British Journal of Dermatology*, vol. 94, no. 4, pp. 401–6.
10. Price, W., 2010, 'Plants bite back: The surprising, all-natural anti-nutrients and toxins in plant foods', *Sign of the Times*, retrieved from: www.sott.net
11. Williams, G.D. et.al., 2011, 'Salicylate intoxication from teething gel in infancy', *Med J Aust*, 194(3), pp. 146–8.
12. ibid.
13. Loblay, R.H. and Swain, A.R., 2006.
14. ibid.
15. Onyema, O.O. et al., 2006, 'Effect of vitamin E on monosodium glutamate induced hepatotoxicity and oxidative stress in rats', *Indian Journal of Biochemistry and Biophysics*, vol. 43, pp. 20–4.
16. Loblay, R.H. and Swain, A.R., 2006.
17. Cordain, L., et al., 2005, 'Origins and evolution of the western diet: Health implications for the 21st century', *American Journal of Clinical Nutrition*, vol. 81, pp. 341–54.
18. Loblay, R.H. and Swain, A.R., 2006.
19. Dengate, S., 2007, 'Dangers of dried fruit', Food Intolerance Network Factsheet, retrieved from: fedup.com.au
20. Loblay, R.H. and Swain, A.R., 2006.
21. Gupta, C., et al., 2010, 'Antioxidant and antimutagenic effect of quercetin against DEN induced hepatotoxicity in rat', *Phytotherapy Research*, vol. 24, no. 1, pp. 119–28.
22. Garc Roché, M.O., 2006, 'Effect of ascorbic acid on the hepatotoxicity due to the daily intake of nitrate, nitrite and dimethylamine', *Food/Nahrung*, vol. 31, no. 2, pp. 99–104.
23. Jerome, J.J. et al., 1976, 'Inhibition of amine-nitrite hepatotoxicity by α-toco-pherol', *Toxicology and Applied Pharmacology*, vol. 41, no. 3, pp. 575–83.
24. Choi, H., Schmidbauer, N., Sundell, J., Hasselgren, M., Spengler, J. and Bornehag, C.G., 2010, 'Common household chemicals and the allergy risks in pre-school age children', *PLoS One*, 5(10), p.e13423.
25. ibid.
26. Chung, Y.M., Kim, B.S., Kim, N.I., Lee, E.Y. and Choue, R., 2005, 'Study of nutritional status, dietary patterns, and dietary quality of atopic dermatitis patients', *Korean Journal of Nutrition*, 38(6), pp. 419–31.
27. ibid.
28. Sydenstricker, V.P., et al., 1942, 'Observations on the "egg white injury" in man and its cure with a biotin concentrate', *Journal of the American Medical Association*, vol. 118, no. 14, pp. 1199–200.
29. Pasmans, S.G., Preesman, A.H. and Van Vloten, W.A., 1998. 'Pellagra (deficiency of vitamin B3 or of the amino acid tryptophan): A disease still extant in the Netherlands', *Nederlands Tijdschrift Vor Geneeskunde*, vol. 142, no. 33, pp. 1880–2.
30. Swain, A.R., Dutton, S.P. and Truswell, A.S., 1985, 'Salicylates in foods', *J Am Diet Assoc*, 85(8), pp. 950–60, retrieved from: http://www.slhd.nsw.gov.au/rpa/allergy/research/salicylatesinfoods.pdf
31. ibid.
32. ibid.
33. Uenishi, T., Sugiura, H. and Uehara, M., 2003, 'Role of foods in irregular aggravation of atopic dermatitis', *Journal of Dermatology*, vol. 30, pp. 91–7.
34. Swain, A.R., Dutton, S.P. and Truswell, A.S., 1985.
35. ibid.
36. ibid.
37. ibid.
38. Micha, R., Michas, G. and Mozaffarian, D., 2012, 'Unprocessed red and processed meats and risk of coronary artery disease and type 2 diabetes: An updated review of the evidence', *Current atherosclerosis reports*, 14(6), pp. 515–24.
39. Sydenstricker, V.P., et al., 1942, 'Observations on the "egg white injury" in man and its cure with a biotin concentrate', *Journal of the American Medical Association*, vol. 118, no. 14, pp. 1199–200.
40. Oracz, J. and Nebesny, E., 2014, 'Influence of roasting conditions on the biogenic amine content in cocoa beans of different Theobroma cacao cultivars,' *Food Research International*, vol. 55, pp. 1–10.
41. Isolauri, E. and Turjanmaa, K., 1996, 'Combined skin prick and patch testing enhances

identification of food allergy in infants with atopic dermatitis', *Journal of Allergy and Clinical Immunology*, 97(1), pp. 9–15.

3. Before you begin: do this now

1. Maintz, L. and Novak, N., 2007, 'Histamine and histamine intolerance', *American Journal of Clinical Nutrition*, vol. 85, no. 5, pp. 1185–96.
2. ibid.

4. Choose your program

1. Beath, S.V., 2003, 'Hepatic function and physiology in the newborn', in *Seminars in Neonatology*, vol. 8, no. 5, pp. 337–46.
2. Kimata, H., 2005, 'Prevalence of fatty liver in non-obese Japanese children with atopic dermatitis', *Indian Pediatrics*, vol. 42, no. 6, p. 587.
3. Loblay, R.H. and Swain, A.R., 2006.
4. 'Fibrous degeneration of connective tissue caused by excessive acidity in the body', in *Mosby's Medical Dictionary*, 10th edition, 2017
5. Brocard, A., Quereux, G., Moyse, D. and Dreno, B., 2010, 'Localized scleroderma and zinc: A pilot study', *European Journal of Dermatology*, 20(2), pp. 172–4.
6. Namazi, M.R. and Leok, G.C., 2009, 'Vitiligo and diet: A theoretical molecular approach with practical implications', *Indian Journal of Dermatology, Venereology, and Leprology*, 75(2), p. 116.

5. Top 12 foods for eliminating eczema

1. Zeisel, S.H. et al., 2003, 'Concentrations of choline-containing compounds and betaine in common foods', *Journal of Nutrition*, 133(5), pp. 1302–7.
2. Hix, L. et al., 2004, 'Bioactive carotenoids: Potent antioxidants and regulators of gene expression', *Redox Report*, vol. 9, no. 4, pp. 181–91.
3. Khazdair, M.R. et al., 2015, 'The effects of Crocus sativus (saffron) and its constituents on nervous system: A review', *Avicenna Journal of Phytomedicine*, vol. 5, no. 5, p. 376.

6. Other useful ingredients

1. Sausenthaler, S. et al., 2006, 'Margarine and butter consumption, eczema and allergic sensitization in children', *Pediatric Allergy and Immunology*, vol. 17, no. 2, pp. 85–93.
2. Bolte, G, et al., 2001, 'Margarine consumption and allergy in children', *American Journal of Respiratory and Critical Care Medicine*, vol. 163, pp. 277–9.
3. Sausenthaler, S., et al., 2007, 'Maternal diet during pregnancy in relation to eczema and allergic sensitization in the offspring at 2 years of age', *American Journal of Clinical Nutrition*, vol. 85, pp. 530–7.

7. Skin Supplement Program

1. Cabrini, L., Bergami, R., Fiorentini, D., Marchetti, M., Landi, L. and Tolomelli, B., 1998, 'Vitamin B6 deficiency affects antioxidant defences in rat liver and heart', *IUBMB Life*, 46(4), pp. 689–97.
2. Marone, G. et al., 1986, 'Physiological concentrations of zinc inhibit the release of histamine from human basophils and lung mast cells', *Agents and Actions*, 18(1–2), pp. 103–6.
3. De Spirt, S. et al., 2009, 'Intervention with flaxseed and borage oil supplements modulates skin condition in women', *British Journal of Nutrition*, vol. 101, pp. 440–45.
4. Simopoulos, A.P., 2002, 'The importance of the ratio of omega-6/omega-3 essential fatty acids', *Biomedicine & Pharmacotherapy*, 56(8), pp. 365–79.
5. Zhang, C.G. and Kim, S.J., 2007, 'Taurine induces anti-anxiety by activating strychnine-sensitive glycine receptor in vivo', *Annals of Nutrition and Metabolism*, vol. 51, no. 4, pp. 379–86.
6. National Center for Biotechnology Information. PubChem compound database; CID=1123, https://pubchem.ncbi.nlm.nih.gov/compound/1123.
7. ibid.
8. Liu, Y. et al., 1998, 'Taurine chloramine inhibits production of nitric oxide and prostaglandin E 2 in activated C6 glioma cells by suppressing inducible nitric oxide synthase and cyclooxygenase-2 expression', *Molecular Brain Research*, vol. 59, no. 2, pp. 189–95.
9. Gentile, C.L. et al., 2011, 'Experimental evidence for therapeutic potential of taurine in the treatment of non-alcoholic fatty liver disease', *American Journal of Physiology-Regulatory, Integrative and Comparative Physiology*, vol. 301, no. 6, pp. R1710–22.
10. Kimata, H., 2005, 'Prevalence of fatty liver in non-obese Japanese children with atopic dermatitis', *Indian Pediatrics*, vol. 42, no. 6, p. 587.
11. Papaioannou, R. and Pfeiffer, C.C., 1984, 'Sulfite sensitivity-unrecognized threat: Is molybdenum deficiency the cause?' *Journal of Orthomolecular Psychiatry*, 13(2), pp. 105–10.
12. Abumrad, N.N., 1984, 'Molybdenum — is it an essential trace metal?' *Bulletin of the New York Academy of Medicine*, 60(2), p. 163.
13. ibid.
14. Papaioannou, R. and Pfeiffer, C.C., 1984.
15. Abumrad, N.N., 1984.

8. Food Intolerance Diagnosis (FID) Program

1. Loblay, R.H. and Swain, A.R., 2006.
2. Manach, C. et al., 2004, 'Polyphenols: Food sources and bioavailability', *American Journal of Clinical Nutrition*, 79(5), pp. 727–47.
3. Serrano, J. et al., 2009, 'Tannins: Current knowledge of food sources, intake, bioavailability and biological effects', *Molecular Nutrition & Food Research*, 53(S2), pp. S310–29.
4. Swain, A.R., Dutton, S.P. and Truswell, A.S., 1985, 'Salicylates in foods', *J Am Diet Assoc*, 85(8), pp. 950–60.
5. Loblay, R.H. and Swain, A.R., 2006.
6. ibid.

9. Eczema Detox Program and menus

1. Loblay, R.H. and Swain, A.R., 2006, 'Food Intolerance', *Recent Advances in Clinical Nutrition*, retrieved 1 October 2016 retrieved from: www.nsw.gov.au.
2. Swain, A.R., Dutton, S.P. and Truswell, A.S., 1985.
3. Manach, C. et al., 2004.
4. Serrano, J. et al., 2009, 'Tannins: Current knowledge of food sources, intake, bioavailability and biological effects', *Molecular Nutrition & Food Research*, 53(S2), pp. S310–29.

11. Babies with eczema

1. Williams, G.D. et al., 2011, 'Salicylate intoxication from teething gel in infancy', *Med J Aust*, 194(3), pp. 146–8.

12. FAQs and problem solving

1. Isolauri, E. and Turjanmaa, K., 1996, 'Combined skin prick and patch testing enhances identification of food allergy in infants with atopic dermatitis', *Journal of Allergy and Clinical Immunology*, 97(1), pp. 9–15.
2. Loblay, R.H. and Swain, A.R., 2006.
3. Dengate, S., 2016, 'What's wrong with potatoes?' *Food Intolerance Network*, retrieved from: www.fedup.com.au
4. Source: Swain, A.R., Dutton, S.P. and Truswell, A.S. 1985, 'Salicylates in foods', *Journal of the American Dietetic Association*, vol. 85, no. 8, pp.950–60.

Recipe index

Index